DATE DUE

T R

THE EXCIMER

Fundamentals and Clinical Use

Second Edition

Harold A. Stein, MD, FRCS(C)
Albert T. Cheskes, MD, FRCS(C)
Raymond M. Stein, MD, FRCS(C)

SLACK Incorporated, 6900 Grove Road, Thorofare, NJ 08086-9447

5/00

Note to the Reader

Any book about an emerging trend or technology will have an evolving role in the professional literature. As this book covers the fundamentals of a device recently approved by the Food and Drug Administration in the United States, future developments are to be expected by physicians and researchers throughout the world. The authors and the publisher welcome all suggestions for improvements and inclusion of additional material in future editions of this work.

Publisher: John H. Bond
Editorial Director: Amy E. Drummond
Associate Editor: Jennifer J. Cahill
Creative Director: Linda Baker

The procedures and practices described in this book should be implemented in a manner consistent with the professional standards set for the circumstances that apply in each specific situation. Every effort has been made to confirm the accuracy of the information presented and to correctly relate generally accepted practices. The authors, editor, and publisher cannot accept responsibility for errors or exclusions or for the outcome of the material presented herein. There is no expressed or implied warranty of this book or information imparted by it.

Care has been taken to ensure that drug selection and dosages are in accordance with currently accepted/recommended practice. Due to continuing research, changes in government policy and regulations, and various effects of drug reactions and interactions, it is recommended that the reader carefully review all materials and literature provided for each drug, especially those that are new or not frequently used.

Stein, Harold A.

The excimer: fundamentals and clinical use/ Harold A. Stein, Albert T. Cheskes, Raymond M. Stein--2nd ed.

p. cm.

Includes bibliographical references and index.

ISBN 1-55642-338-1

1. Lasers in ophthalmology. 2. Excimer lasers--Therapeutic use. I. Cheskes, Albert. II. Stein, Raymond M. III. Title.

[DNLM: 1. Keratotomy, Radial. 2. Refractive Errors--surgery. 3. Laser Surgery--methods. WW 220 S819e 1997]

RE86.S74 1997

617.7'55--dc21

DNLM/DLC

for Library of Congress 97-10945

Printed in the United States of America

Published by: SLACK Incorporated
6900 Grove Road
Thorofare, NJ 08086-9447 USA
Telephone: 609-848-1000
Fax: 609-853-5991

Contact SLACK Incorporated for more information about other books in this field or about the availability of our books from distributors outside the United States.

Contents

Acknowledgments

We are indebted to Jill Klintworth, Cindi Price, Ghani A. Salim, Robin Inrig, and Raphael DePhilipo, MD, who have helped us in many aspects of the second edition. They have helped us not only in their dedication to laser treatment, but for their interpersonal skills with patients, which have helped us enjoy success in patient management.

We are again indebted to Maria Aparecida Mesa Munarin, MD, for her early collating reference material for the first edition, and to Mr. Michael W. Malley of the CRM Group for his unique, creative method of marketing and his presentation in this book.

We would also like to thank Mr. Robert Shropshire of MAD Dog Communications for professional marketing, which has helped our practice grow.

Contributors

Harold A. Stein, MD, FRCS(C)
Professor of Ophthalmology, University of Toronto; Attending
Ophthalmologist, Mt. Sinai Hospital and Scarborough General Hospital,
Toronto, Ontario; Past President, Contact Lens Association of
Ophthalmologists, New Orleans, Louisiana; Past President, Canadian
Ophthalmologic Society, Ottawa; Past President, Joint
Commission on Allied Health Personnel in Ophthalmology, St. Paul,
Minnesota; Director, Bochner Eye Institute, Toronto, Ontario, Canada.

Albert T. Cheskes, MD, FRCS(C)
Chief, Department of Ophthalmology, Centenary Health Centre, Toronto;
Assistant Professor, Department of Ophthalmology, University of
Toronto; Attending Ophthalmologist, Wellesley Central Hospital and
Sunnybrook Hospital, Toronto, Ontario; Past Chairman, Eye
Safety Committee, Canadian Ophthalmologic Society; Member, Mayo
Clinic, Ophthalmology Alumni, Rochester, Minnesota; Consultant,
Bochner Eye Institute, Toronto, Ontario, Canada.

Raymond M. Stein, MD, FRCS(C)
Chief of Ophthalmology, Scarborough General Hospital, Toronto, Ontario;
Assistant Professor, Department of Ophthalmology, University of
Toronto; Medical Consultant, Beacon Eye Institute, Toronto, Ontario;
Cornea Consultant, Mt. Sinai Hospital, Central Hospital, and Bochner Eye
Institute, Toronto, Ontario, Canada; Director, Mayo Clinic, Ophthalmology
Alumni, Rochester, Minnesota; Past Commissioner, Joint Commission on
Allied Health Personnel in Ophthalmology, St. Paul, Minnesota; Member,
Eye Safety Committee, Canadian Ophthalmologic Society.

Foreword

It is no coincidence that the first clinically detailed excimer text has been prepared by three Canadian authors who are early users of an American manufactured excimer system. While the Food and Drug Administration (FDA) regulations in the United States restricted the use of the excimer in the country of its invention to a limited number of patients, the less rigid Canadian regulatory environment allowed a more rapid appreciation and development of the clinical value of this technology.

Canadian surgeons adopted excimer lasers to treat refractive errors with enthusiasm, none more so than those at the Maxwell K. Bochner Eye Institute in Toronto. The authors, Harold A. Stein, Albert T. Cheskes, and Raymond M. Stein, pioneers in the Canadian excimer program, received their laser system in September 1991. They have 3 years of practical experience in an outpatient clinical environment using excimer lasers to treat myopic refractive errors. This group has had substantial previous experience with refractive surgery and is able to make a fair comparison between the results that are obtained with the excimer laser and results using other refractive technologies.

There is value in carefully constructed long-term clinical studies of limited populations such as those that are required by the FDA. There is also substantial value to reports from clinical practitioners working in the intimate doctor/patient relationship who offer this service in the anticipation of an excellent result. The three authors of this book are in this position and have worked long and hard to meet the expectations of their patients. We will all benefit from their manifold observations of patient selection, management, and the many surgical details which can only be learned with a large volume of clinical experience.

There is much to learn, and there is no doubt that the clinical work of Canadian surgeons has made the path to be followed less difficult for all of us.

Stephen L. Trokel, MD
Harkness Eye Institute
New York, New York
October 1994

Preface to the Second Edition

Refractive surgery is now a subspecialty and has become a major clinical thrust in ophthalmology since our first edition was published. Many scientific articles, textbooks, and presentations have appeared to the scientific community. The public is also well informed with considerable information available on the Internet.

A major shift in medical, media, and public attitude has occurred regarding the human ability to alter the normal eye to improve uncorrected visual acuity. As a by-product of this technology, there has been an expansion of its therapeutic application in altering the corneal surface to restore sight.

At the time of this writing, the excimer laser has obtained limited approval in the United States. Undoubtedly, this will expand. As well, new foreign excimer laser companies will appear on the scene. These are based on scanning systems with slit or spot type as compared to the broad beam of VisX and Summit. All eyecare practitioners must be prepared for the coming refractive revolution. We now have tremendous, highly sophisticated tools that were unheard of a decade ago.

This book remains true to its original mission: to present an easy-to-read book on basics and clinical information about the excimer laser in photorefractive keratectomy (PRK). Of new and increasing popularity is the role of Laser Assisted In Situ Keratomileusis (LASIK) along with a few newer alternatives in refractive surgery. A chapter on LASIK has been added, along with expanded discussion of other options. For those seeking details in these areas, the reader should consult other texts and the scientific literature.

We have added more details on new excimer laser models found in the international arena. We have added clinical material on new laser ablation techniques and postoperative management. For this we have called upon experiences at both the Bochner Eye Institute and the Beacon Eye Institute. We have added tables, figures, and opinions from many of our distinguished colleagues who have made and continue to make fine contributions to the exciting field of excimer laser technology.

Preface to the First Edition

This book is written for the general ophthalmologist who does not yet have an excimer laser and wishes to begin the process of incorporating refractive surgery into his or her practice. It is also directed to the optometrist and other eyecare practitioners who wish to have an understanding of the processes involved in the use of the excimer laser and the state of excimer laser technology today.

Obviously, excimer laser technology will change rapidly. However, we have tried to encompass the current state-of-the-art of some of the major areas of excimer laser technology. Patients are now well aware of this technological breakthrough and will be demanding information on this process.

We have tried as much as possible to introduce some of our own experiences and practical management of the typical patient vis-à-vis the excimer laser. We have been involved in radial keratotomy (RK) for the past 10 years but have now shifted our emphasis to laser technology, which appears to be on the cutting edge of refractive surgery.

Most refractive surgery procedures require a long learning curve. Such is also the case with the excimer laser. The procedural portion of the learning curve can be relatively short. However, there are many nuances in the treatment and management of patients that we feel compelled to introduce from our experience.

There are many laser unknowns still present. We do not know how deep we can do ablations without creating descemetoceles. We do not know its impact on keratoconus—will it help or harm? Will it correct irregular as well as regular astigmatism so that a contact lens can be worn? We do not know the risks of decreased best-corrected vision. We do not know the regression rate of high myopia treatments. Hyperopia treatment is just developing. We do not yet know its efficacy. How many times can we remove haze from subsequent reablations? If we overshoot or undershoot the mark, can we reverse it by modulating drops or further excimer treatment? Do we know all the risks?

As information expands worldwide, we feel privileged to be part of the information explosion.

Introduction to the First Edition

In the 1990s the ophthalmic community is making a concerted effort to correct refractive errors and restore normal uncorrected vision to 20/20. There are more than 75 million myopic patients in North America in addition to the 25 million contact lens wearers. More than 90% of the refractive errors that require correction are <6 D.

This is the decade in which the population will be heavily marketed to have a lifestyle free of spectacles and contact lenses. Occupations such as firefighters, police officers, etc., already have a sight requirement for admission because of safety considerations. However, lifestyle improvement is probably the single largest factor that causes patients to seek correction of their refractive errors. The move to throw away glasses and contact lenses has been ushered in by recent criticism in the journals about contact lenses. The safety of contact lenses has been challenged in many articles, but probably most importantly by the *New England Journal of Medicine* of September 21, 1989, which reported that corneal ulcers occurred 9 to 13 times more often with extended wear lenses. Corneal ulceration starts with micro-trauma of the cornea permitting small portals of entry caused by hypoxia under the contact lens. Through these tiny portals microorganisms can then invade the cornea. Corneal ulcers have been reported to occur in 30% of cases secondary to lens wear.

Another problem with contact lenses has been down-time. The individual may have minor irritations which will not permit him or her to wear contact lenses. He or she must return to the workforce wearing spectacles. In addition to contact lens intolerance, there are many individuals who are too nervous to insert anything into their eyes. These people are ideal candidates for the PRK procedure with the excimer laser. There will be several thousand ophthalmologists and optometrists involved in some aspect of identifying patients for PRK once the excimer laser has been approved in the United States. In those parts of the world where PRK has been introduced, such as Canada, Europe, and Asia, the PRK procedure has enjoyed great success. As more patients undergo PRK and spread the word of success, more candidates will begin to seek this procedure. It has been estimated that there will be 3 to 4 million PRK procedures performed annually at a cost of $1500 to $2500 per eye. PRK could become one of the most exciting and interesting new procedures performed in this decade, and could create a large financial and employment growth in industry as well. There are currently more than 500 excimer lasers for PRK that have been installed worldwide since 1988. More than 300,000 eyes have been treated at the time of this writing. The 1-year clinical results from the major laser manufacturers show refractive stability after 6 to 9 months and achieved corrections of ±1 D of emmetropia for at least 80% of patients, and significantly more have achieved +1.5 D to -1.5 D of emmetropia.

There is certainly no question that the excimer laser works. It will have a major impact on the delivery of eyecare and will become the most user-friendly of all the refractive procedures to date. Whether the number of patients who are going to have excimer laser treatment performed is overestimated or even underestimated, no one will know until approval in the United States and large-scale marketing has run its course. However, we do know that this procedure will become shared among eyecare providers and there will be ongoing management of patients. There are many models of comanagement in which the optometrist and ophthalmologist can come together and share their expertise in the management of refractive errors. Centers will undoubtedly spring up throughout North America as laser manufacturers gear up for sale to a large market. Fifty percent of the world market is in the United States, which contains perhaps the most affluent population in the world. The United States also houses the largest media groups in the world, which can have a profound influence on the lives of millions of people.

The excimer laser will certainly affect the lives of those who will be able to change their vocation or avocation, or be of help to them with skiing, swimming, and other sporting events, as well as their lifestyle. Of significant benefit will be its therapeutic use, which can bring sight to many and spare the need for corneal transplantation with the attendant risks of an invasive procedure.

RK currently is the most-performed refractive surgery in the United States. The major advantages of PRK over RK are that it leaves a structurally sound eye and is not as operator dependent. PRK relies on a computer for its accuracy and predictability and not the human hand. As RK candidates are given the option for PRK, the demand for laser surgery will certainly explode in North America as it has in Canada in the past few years.

What is unique about the excimer laser is that it has strong acceptance by our peers, by the public, and by all eyecare providers. Unlike most other refractive procedures, there is no antagonism toward PRK because it does not invade what was considered a normal cornea. The word laser equals high safety and high technology. It is a buzzword for individuals who have followed laser treatments in many other areas of medicine and have associated it with high success.

Generating even more enthusiasm is the precision of the excimer laser. The development of an innovative machine, the videokeratoscope, has allowed much more sophisticated analysis of how the cornea is shaped and what is happening to the cornea after any procedure. Topographic analysis of the cornea with this device has greatly increased our ability to evaluate and improve the PRK procedure.

Such technological advancements will go hand in hand with new innovations in the excimer laser itself, constantly improving the procedure. As PRK and other ophthalmic applications of the excimer laser are performed in greater numbers, its efficacy and safety will continue to be improved and costs will be reduced, allowing even more people to enjoy the advantages of treatment with the excimer laser.

Harold A. Stein, MD, FRCS(C)
Albert T. Cheskes, MD, FRCS(C)
Raymond M. Stein, MD, FRCS(C)

Basics

Chapter 1

Basics of Excimer Laser Technology and History

Facts on Lasers

Basics of General Laser Physics

- The word *laser* stands for light amplification by stimulated emission of radiation.
- Electromagnetic radiation contains two properties which are wave- and particle-like.
- Electron orbitals consist of clouds of electrons. These orbitals have different energy levels and surround the protons and neutrons which make up the nucleus of an atom. An atom in its ground state of energy (lowest level) absorbs external energy (Figure 1-1) through the electrons moving from lower level orbitals, which have less energy, to higher level orbitals. When the electron moves from a higher level orbital back to its ground state, a photon of energy (wave) is produced. This process is known as spontaneous emission.
- When electrons are moved to this higher energy level by outside forces, nearby atoms may also begin to elevate to higher levels, emitting waves or photons in phase with each other. The waves add energy to one another and create a high energy beam of laser light.

Characteristics of the Laser Light

- **Brightness**—the measurement of energy for the laser beam is radiant exposure (energy/unit area), also known as fluence (mJ/cm^2).
- **Coherence**—pertains to waves with a continuous relationship among phases. It is created by the geometry of the resonant cavity of the laser. Spatial coherence describes where the "peaks and valleys" occur in the

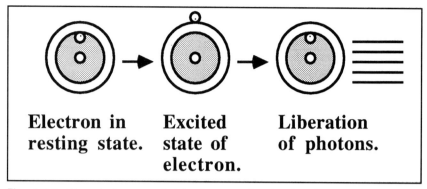

Figure 1-1. Atoms in the ground state of energy absorb external energy through electrons moving from lower to higher level orbitals.

laser beam. The regularity of spatial coherence depends on the laser's monochromaticity and directionality and is primarily caused by the geometry of the laser. When a wavelength does not change in time, it is known as temporal coherence.

- **Directionality**—the laser beam is able to be directed at a very small area quite a distance from the laser itself. The directionality is measured by the full angle beam divergence in radians.

- **Emission of the Laser Light**—the distribution of energy in a laser beam is the mode of the beam. The energy perpendicular to the direction of the beam is the transverse mode and the energy along the same direction as the laser beam is the longitudinal mode. The transverse electromagnetic mode (TEM) depends on the laser cavity. The simpler the mode structure, the more homogeneous the beam. If there is more power in the center of the beam than at the edge, the mode is designated TEM. Laser beams can acquire many mode structures, in which case it is called multimode.

- **Types of Emission**—laser light can be emitted either continuously or in pulses (Figure 1-2). With continuous wave lasers, a constant pumping of the laser medium leads to a stationary emission of light, such as in the familiar argon laser. With pulsed lasers, such as the excimer laser, excitation of the laser medium is achieved by single events, such as an electrical discharge, leading to a single, short emission of light, the laser pulse. The pulsed laser is approximately 1000 to 1,000,000 times more powerful than a continuous wave laser. Only pulsed lasers are useful in refractive corneal surgery.

- **Monochromaticity**—a characteristic of the laser which contains a single wavelength of light.

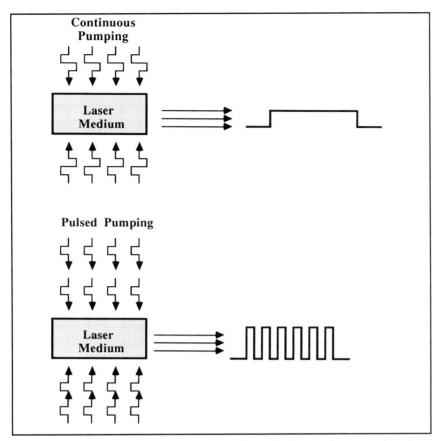

Figure 1-2. The laser beam may be a wave form that is continuous or in pulses. Modified from Waring GO. *Trans Am Ophthalmol Soc.* 1989;87:854-983.

Laser Interactions

- The term *excimer* comes from the words *excited* and *dimer*. *Excited dimer* means two atoms which exist only in an excited state. When electronically excited, two atoms form one stable molecule. In the excimer, this is a combination of a halogen and an insert gas. These do not combine easily (Figure 1-3). The atoms must be elevated to a high energy state, which requires high voltage and high power discharge into the gaseous mixture. There is almost no absorption at this state. This lack of absorption results in high power and short energy pulses.

Delivery of the Laser

- Devices such as circular diaphragms, rotating slits, or contact masks should be used to make the beam circular because the energy created cannot be focused to one point. Depending on the optics of the delivery system, the beam created is broad and rectangular.

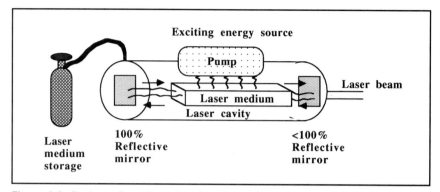

Figure 1-3. Basic configuration of excimer laser demonstrates the active laser medium as gas in the storage tank and in the laser cavity. The excited energy is pumped from a source illustrated as a bank of electrical capacitors whose discharge can create a population inversion in the laser medium. The laser cavity has mirrors at each end to amplify the laser beam before it is emitted through a delivery system containing lenses. Modified from Waring GO. *Trans Am Ophthalmol Soc.* 1989;87:854-983.

• Each pulse of the excimer laser destroys a specific amount of tissue.

Multiple pulses destroy deeper layers; each pulse removes approximately 0.25 µm of corneal tissue.

The optical delivery system differs according to brand. A uniform beam profile can be produced with the beam shaping and beam homogenizing optics. The iris beam delivery system (Figure 1-4) is present in VisX Inc (Santa Clara, California), Nidek Inc (Fremont, California), and Summit Technology (Waltham, Massachusetts) lasers. The Aesculap-Meditec (Jena, Germany) lasers use a scanning beam, in which the iris diaphragm is supported by a suction ring fixed on the patient's eye.

In the excimer laser, specialized ultraviolet (UV)-grade optical elements must be used, as the far UV photons are quite damaging to normal glass elements. In ophthalmic excimer lasers, the delivery system is made coaxial with an operating microscope so that the surgeon can visualize directly the effects on the cornea.

All of the ophthalmic excimer lasers are controlled by computers; energy levels, pulse rates, and other parameters can be preprogrammed. Some of the lasers also have videocameras and screen monitors.

Laser/Tissue Interactions

Photoablative decomposition is the clean and precise removal of corneal tissue with the excimer laser. This occurs when far UV radiation reacts with protein molecules, resulting in the photochemical breakage of the molecular bonds with no local thermal effect (Figure 1-5). The source of the far UV photons is a high efficiency gas discharge excimer laser which

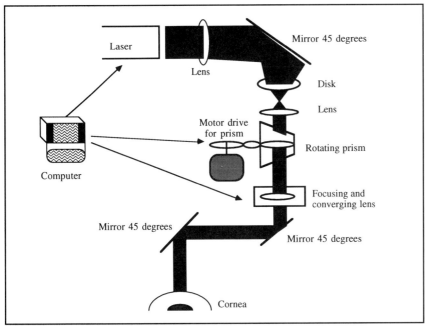

Figure 1-4. Example of excimer laser delivery system. The major components of the IBM computer-controlled, translating slit delivery system. The laser beam is expanded by a lens and diverted toward the eye through a series of mirrors. It passes through the calibrated slit mask, and the image of the slit is passed through a rotating dove prism that can change the orientation of the slit under computer control. The objective lens moves in the x, y, and z directions under computer control and moves the slit image over the surface of the cornea. Modified from Hanna KD, Chastan JC, Asfar L, et al. *J Cataract Refract Surg.* 1989;15:390-396.

electronically excites a combination of a rare gas (argon) and the halogen (fluorine). This combination produces a laser wavelength of 193 nanometers (nm) in the far UV range (Figure 1-6).

- Excimer lasers produce short, concentrated pulses, removing approximately 0.25 μm of tissue per pulse.
- Penetration can be extremely predictable regarding depth and target zone.

In addition to treating myopia and astigmatism, new developments in hyperopic modules are being developed and will be discussed in Chapter 12.

History of the Excimer Laser in Ophthalmology

The concept of rare gas dimers such as xenon and krypton had been suggested by individuals such as James Keck at the Avco Everett Research Laboratory as early as the 1960s. Excimer laser technology was developed at IBM in 1976, and has been used in industry for many years. Excimers

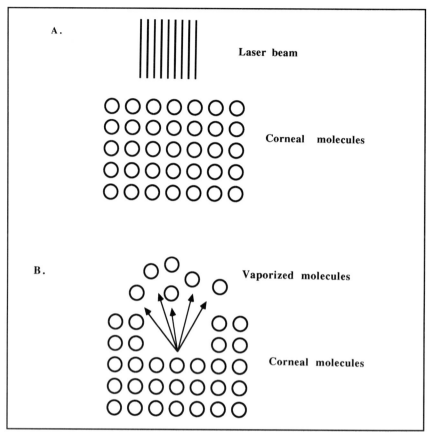

Figure 1-5. (A) PRK with the excimer laser is possible because of the high energy of the laser beam. (B) The laser results in the breakage of intermolecular bonds and the vaporization of molecules leaving the underlying surface relatively unaffected.

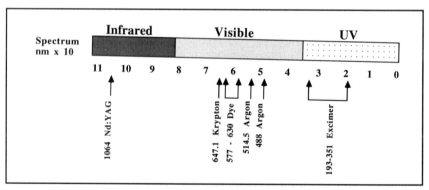

Figure 1-6. Frequency of the near infrared, visible, and UV portions of the electromagnetic spectrum with various lasers.

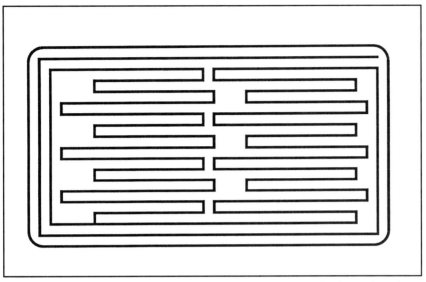

Figure 1-7. An illustration of a microchip that has been etched by the excimer laser. Note the detail and precision of the ablation.

have the desirable qualities of producing very precise destruction with almost negligible effects outside the target zone. For this reason, these lasers have been used extensively in the creation of sophisticated computer microchips (Figure 1-7, Table 1-1).

In the early 1980s, Srinivasan and colleagues at IBM demonstrated that UV radiation from the argon fluoride (ArF) excimer laser was able to precisely etch (to the submicron level) synthetic and organic polymers.

In 1981, the excimer laser was shown to have an effect on superficial corneal tissue. In the first publication to describe this application, Tabaoda, Mikesell, and Reed showed that corneal epithelium is extremely sensitive to the 193-nm light emitted by the ArF excimer laser.

In June 1983, Stephen L. Trokel collaborated with Srinivasan, a physicist at the IBM Thomas J. Watson Research Center in Yorktown Heights, New York. This work showed that the cornea of a bovine eye responded to excimer laser radiation while the adjacent tissue suffered no thermal damage. Trokel received a patent in 1983 based on the experiments on bovine corneas.

A Lambda Physic excimer laser was later installed at the Edward S. Harkness Eye Institute at the Columbia-Presbyterian Medical Center, and numerous experiments with rabbit and monkey eyes were conducted. This multimillion-dollar commitment, involving investors, multiple patents, and the recruitment of physicists, engineers, and medical personnel, introduced

Table 1-1.
Introduction of the Excimer Laser

Year	Event
1976	Developed and used by IBM for computer microchips
1981	First publication by Tabaoda, Mikesell, and Reed
1983	Landmark report in ophthalmic literature by Trokel, Srinivasan, and Braren
1983	Trokel publication with bovine cornea
1985	First human eye treated by Seiler in Berlin
1986	First normal sighted eye treated by Seiler
1988	First normal sighted eye treated by McDonald in North America

Table 1-2.
Ophthalmic Lasers: First Clinical Use

Year	Laser	Clinician
1963	Ruby	Campbell, Zweng
1968	Argon	L'Esperance
1971	Frequency-doubled Nd:YAG	L'Esperance
1972	Krypton	L'Esperance
1972	Carbon dioxide	L'Esperance
1973	Nd:YAG (CW)	Beckman
1977	Nd:YAG (mode-locked)	Aron-Rosa
1979	Dye (Q-switched)	Bass
1981	Dye (CW)	L'Esperance
1981	Nd:YAG (Q-switched)	Fankhauser
1985	Excimer laser	Seiler, Wollensak

Modified from L'Esperance FA. Ophthalmic lasers. 3rd ed. 1989.

the utilization of the excimer laser for experimental and clinical evaluation.

The first clinical application of the excimer laser was by Theo Seiler in Berlin in April 1985 (Table 1-2). He initiated a study of linear incisions using his contact mask technique followed by the creation of transverse incisions (T-cuts) in September 1985 to correct astigmatism in blind human eyes. One month later, Seiler performed the first excimer refractive surgery in a sighted eye with a malignant melanoma scheduled for enucleation. This early work was presented at the German Ophthalmological Society in September 1986.

Also in 1986, Cooper Surgical began to construct an ophthalmic excimer laser system, directed by Charles Munnerlyn, prior to the sale of the Cooper Surgical division to the Alcon Corporation. The new entity became a public company under the name VisX and proceeded to develop its instrumentation and file for the various stages of Food and Drug Administration (FDA) approval.

The first normal sighted eye was ablated by Seiler on January 14, 1987, and his experience was summarized to include the effects upon the corneal curvature of T-cuts in both impaired and normally sighted eyes.

Munnerlyn and coworkers then developed a computer-generated algorithm relating diameter and depth of the ablation to the required dioptric change. These calculations assume that the posterior surface of the cornea remains fixed and that only the anterior surface of the cornea is modified.

Between 1987 and 1989, three companies (Summit Technology, Taunton Technologies, and VisX) were working toward premarket approval to use the ArF excimer laser. Trokel received the first investigational device exemption (IDE) from the FDA to establish clinical trials in phase I studies on human blind eyes or eyes scheduled for enucleation.

Marguerite B. McDonald verified the theoretical basis of photorefractive keratectomy (PRK) in an extensive series of experiments involving rabbits and primates that led to the first successful application in a normally sighted eye in 1987. In 1990, Taunton Technologies acquired VisX, retaining the VisX name.

Excimer laser technology has continued to evolve with the development of scanning and flying spot lasers. Clinical studies have shown that these delivery systems can successfully treat myopia, astigmatism, and hyperopia. Broad beam excimer lasers have improved with the introduction of multipass and multizone techniques to create a smoother ablation. Further studies are necessary to determine which laser delivery system will produce the best clinical results.

Today excimer lasers are being placed in countries throughout the world and are revolutionizing our thinking about the correction of refractive errors.

Chapter 2

Current Internationally Available Models

Excimer laser technology is rapidly proliferating throughout the world. All types of commercial instruments use the same principle for the reprofiling of the corneal surface. It is based on interaction of excimer laser radiation with the corneal tissue and occurs with submicron precision.

There are a number of companies that make excimer lasers that are distributed worldwide (Table 2-1). In the United States, the FDA has given investigational approval only for the VisX and the Summit Technology lasers. There are a number of companies seeking FDA approval in the United States at the time of this writing. There are also a number of companies trying to develop new lasers with new technological advantages.

Current Models

The two most popular North American lasers are those provided by VisX and Summit Technology. The other lasers, such as those manufactured by Aesculap-Meditec, LaserSight Technologies Inc (Orlando, Florida), Chiron Vision Corp (Claremont, California), Nidek, Autonomous Technologies Corp (Orlando, Florida), and Coherent Medical (Palo Alto, California), will be briefly outlined. The individual who has to make a choice as to his or her preferred model must make an extensive study of all these lasers through the company spokesperson, the literature, and communication with experienced laser users.

Important factors to consider are:
- Size of the optical zone
- Whether an astigmatism module is included
- Whether a hyperopic module is included

Table 2-1.
Manufacturers of Excimer Lasers

Aesculap-Meditec (MEL-60, MEL-70)
Autonomous Technologies (T-PRK)
Chiron Vision (Keracor 116, Keracor 117, Technolas 217 C-LASIK)
Coherent Medical (Schwind Keratom)
LaserSight Technologies (Compak-200 Mini Excimer Laser, LaserScan 2000)
Nidek (EC-5000)
Novatec Laser Systems (LightBlade$_2$)
Photon Data (Scan 190)
Summit Technology (SVS Apex Plus)
Telco (Australian Laser)
VisX (20/20 B, STAR)
WaveLight Laser Technologie (Allegro)

- The homogenicity of the laser beam
- The annual operating expense
- The size of the machine and whether one has the facility to house it
- The reliability and predictability of the machine, which should be reviewed by calling some of the users of the particular manufacturer

The outcome analysis should also be determined by calling some of the laser users to be sure they are achieving predictable and stable results.

There are three significant approaches to the mechanism of action. Ronald Krueger has grouped these into hardware similarities and differences. There are essentially three major subgroups:

1. The wide field approach
2. The scanning slit approach
3. The flying spot approach

Below is a summary of their actions and characteristics.

Wide Field (Broad Beam Lasers)

The VisX 20/20 B excimer laser (Figure 2-1) represents a model that is effective for all myopia, including high myopia and myopic astigmatism. It is also effective for astigmatism up to 6 D. The newer and smaller VisX STAR laser is now capable of treating hyperopia. The VisX 20/20 B and STAR will create central islands in approximately 18% of eyes and this has required a prophylactic anti-island software change.

The Summit Technology excimer laser is a much smaller laser that will fit into most ophthalmic office spaces (Figure 2-2). There are ablatable masks which may be used to achieve astigmatic and hyperopic correction. These are still in the investigational stages. The masks were previously

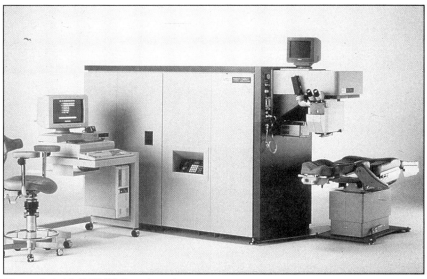

Figure 2-1. VisX 20/20 B excimer laser.

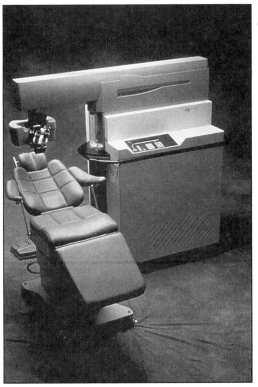

Figure 2-2. Summit Technology excimer laser.

partitioned to the eye but now are positioned in a rail system (Table 2-2).

The original Summit Technology excimer had a small optical zone and did not permit blending of the peripheral shoulder or transition zones. In addition, there were some aggressive changes in the diaphragm opening that permitted

Table 2-2.
Wide Field Approach

- Summit Technology (SVS Apex Plus)
- VisX (20/20 B, STAR)
- Chiron Vision (Keracor 116, Keracor 117)
- Coherent Medical (Schwind Keratom)

Advantages
- Shorter operating time (<30 seconds)
- Eye tracking not needed
- Easy myopia and astigmatism correction
- Higher incidence of central islands

Disadvantages
- High output energy needed
- Good beam uniformity needed
- Hyperopia correction more difficult

Unique Hardware Features

	Summit	VisX	Chiron Vision	Coherent
Beam Shaping				
Myopia	Iris diaphragm	Iris diaphragm	Iris diaphragm	Circular aperture*
Astigmatism	Ablatable mask	Opening slit	Sweeping beam	Elliptical aperture*
Hyperopia	Ablatable mask	Rotating slit with eccentric lens beam	Annular sweeping	Annular aperture*
Beam Smoothing	Conventional optics, oscillating beam	Rotating prism integrator, telescopic zoom	Optical integrator	Optical integrator
Beam Size	6.5 mm	6.5 mm	7.0 mm	8.0 mm
Beam Energy Density	80 mJ/cm²	160 mJ/cm²	120 mJ/cm²	Variable <250 mJ/cm²
Pulse Frequency	10 Hz	10 Hz	10 Hz	13 Hz
Beam Tracking	None	None	Active	Passive

*Also fractile mask.
Adapted with permission from Talamo JH, Krueger RR, eds. The excimer manual: a clinician's guide to excimer laser surgery. Boston: Little, Brown and Co; 1997.

possibly a more aggressive wound healing response. The nomogram called initially for an overcorrection and then epithelial hyperplasia occured. The newer Summit Technology lasers have a larger beam size of 6.5 mm to address some of the night vision problems that were occurring with the original model. It was also able to provide a transition zone and anti-island prophylactic treatment program.

The Technolas (Figure 2-3), distributed in North America through Chiron

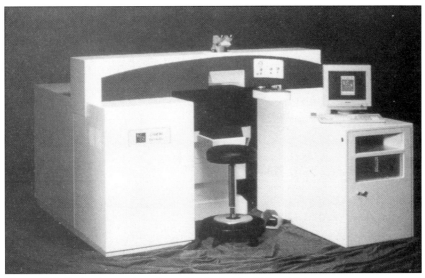

Figure 2-3. Technolas excimer laser distributed by Chiron Vision.

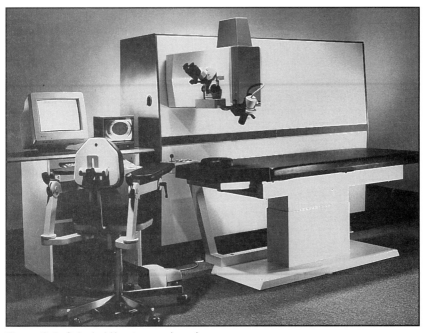

Figure 2-4. Schwind Keratom excimer laser.

Vision, performs ablation for myopia, astigmatism, and hyperopia. It is a microscanning system that eliminates some of the circular grooving seen in some of the wide beam laser models. The 217 C-LASIK incorporates topography into the laser so one can take a corneal map prior to lasing. The new 217 has a 2-mm spot PlanoScan capable of treating myopia, hyperopia, and astigmatism.

The Schwind Keratom laser (Figure 2-4), distributed by Coherent

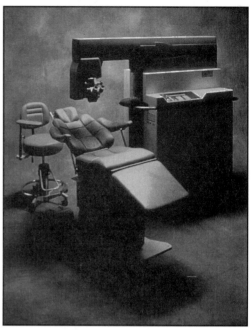

Figure 2-5. Summit Technology Apex Plus model.

Medical, is an ArF excimer laser at 193-nm wavelength. It has a pulse energy of 500 mg (maximum) and a pulse frequency of 13 Hz. A lower pulse visible laser aiming beam marks the optical center of the ablation. There is a maximum diameter of 8 mm.

Scanning Slit Beam

By scanning the treatment area, it becomes very smooth over a broad area and theoretically leads to less haze and less regression. In addition, there is less energy impacted upon the cornea with each shot of the laser. As one increases the treatment zones that are required for hyperopia, one increases the energy delivered to the eye. Scanning beams provide a minimal amount of energy to the tissue with the same effect (Figure 2-5, Table 2-3).

Currently there are 190 Aesculap-Meditec (MEL-60) lasers installed worldwide. The newer laser is the MEL-70. This is a scanning slit laser with a beam profile measuring 1.0 x 10.0 mm. By scanning, the beam covers a wide area of 10.0 x 10.0 mm. They use an aluminum paper method with bright orange backing to perform the fluence test. There is a handpiece designed that adheres to the globe and incorporates the specialized mask. Clinical trials for both hyperopia and presbyopia are currently being performed (Figures 2-6 and 2-7).

The Nidek EC-5000 uses a sweeping beam technology with the beam measuring approximately 2.0 x 7.0 mm. It sweeps across the ablated area several times per cycle changing direction by 30° on each pass with its rotating mirrors. Pulse frequency is variable but ranges from 10 to 50 Hz.

Table 2-3.
Scanning Slit Approach

- Aesculap-Meditec (MEL-60, MEL-70)
- Nidek (EC-5000)

Advantages
- Moderate energy output
- Excellent beam uniformity
- Central island not present
- Fast

Disadvantages
- Eye tracking more important
- Eye-based mask cumbersome (Aesculap-Meditec)

Unique Hardware Features

	Aesculap-Meditec	**Nidek**
Beam Shaping		
Myopia	Rotating hourglass mask	Iris diaphragm with scanning and rotating beam
Astigmatism	Variably rotating hourglass mask	Opening slit with scanning and rotating beam
Hyperopia	Rotating inverse hourglass mask	None
Beam Smoothing	Scanning slit beam	Scanning and rotating rectangle beam
Beam Size	10 x 1.5 mm	7 x 2 mm
Beam Energy Density	250 mJ/cm^2	130 mJ/cm^2
Pulse Frequency	20 Hz	50 Hz (5 scans/sec)
Beam Tracking	None	None

Adapted with permission from Talamo JH, Krueger RR, eds. The excimer manual: a clinician's guide to excimer laser surgery. *Boston: Little, Brown and Co; 1997.*

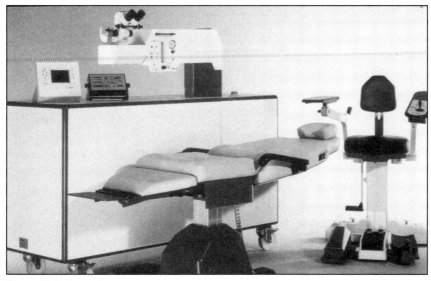

Figure 2-6. Aesculap-Meditec excimer laser.

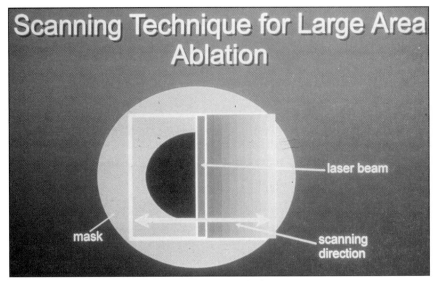

Figure 2-7. Scanning technique for large area ablation.

We are currently using a 46 Hz. The optical zone ranges from 3.0 to 9.0 mm. This permits good transmission zone in the periphery as well as a good delivery for hyperopia from 5.5 to 9.0 mm optical zone. A tracking system is currently being developed.

Nidek laser automatically creates a transition zone between the ablated and unablated corena. It does not require multipass ablation because of the scanning delivery system. Reports from investigators have not found any central islands. The Nidek laser has become our laser of choice for correcting central islands and for removing haze that does not clear with the VisX.

The beam delivery system can be controlled by a three-dimensional motorized joystick and the cornea can be focused by the focus control buttons. Adjust the microscope to the surgeon's pupil distance and magnification to 10X. Adjust the intensity of light. The middle of the two cross-shaped illumination should be aligned to the horizontal center of the pupil by the joystick. The two vertical lines of the cross-shaped illumination on the cornea should be focused to overlap each other at the center by using the focus control.

Both the Aesculap-Meditec and the Nidek can be used for myopia, myopic astigmatism, hyperopia, and hyperopic astigmatism (Figures 2-8 and 2-9).

The Nidek laser is a scanning instrument that eliminates the step process of other broad beam lasers and is said to leave a more uniform surface. Because the Nidek laser can ablate to the 9-mm optical zone, it also has the potential for treating hyperopia.

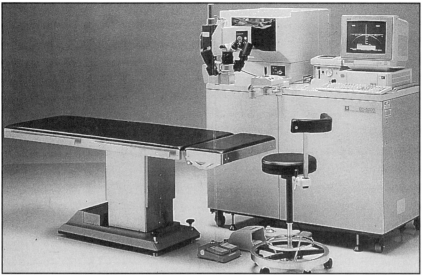

Figure 2-8. Nidek EC-5000 model.

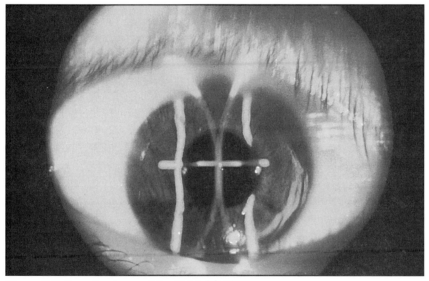

Figure 2-9. Focusing beam of the Nidek EC-5000.

Flying Spot Lasers

Currently there are three flying spot lasers (Table 2-4). The Autonomous Technologies laser currently has only a few lasers operational on the market. Novatec Laser Systems Inc (Carlsbad, California) and the LaserSight Technologies Compak-200 Mini Excimer Laser are achieving some worldwide acceptance in the international market. These lasers represent small energy outputs with lower maintenance cost.

The LaserSight Technologies is a relatively small compact unit. It is

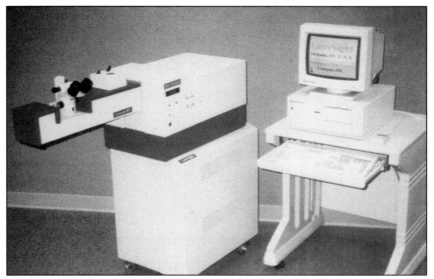

Figure 2-10. Compak-200 Mini Excimer Laser by LaserSight Technologies.

easily portable from office to office. It has a scanning spot and a beam that ranges from 0.8 to 1.2 mm. It has a relatively high pulse rate of 100 Hz. Its main advantage is its uniquely small design and easy installation in small places with fewer optics and automatic gas fill.

The LaserScan 2000 by LaserSight Technologies is the world's smallest PRK laser (Figure 2-10). It has replaced the Mini-200 laser and has fewer optics and automatic gas fill. It has an energy of 2 to 4 mJ, with the fluence on the cornea ranging from 160 to 300 mJ/cm^2. It has an adjustable operating zone of 3 to 9 mm and a computer-controlled scanning mechanism. The scanning system is designed to reduce the risks of uneven ablation and to stop ridges caused by the diaphragm. The constantly moving spot vaporizes a very small area of the stroma as it scans the cornea. It eliminates any unwarranted ridges of the iris diaphragm stop positions. The laser's size is its most significant feature because it provides portability for the laser. It is also low on maintenance and gas costs. It has enhanced software for high myopic correction of up to 15 D using the multizone method. It can also be upgraded for laser thermokeratoplasty (LTK)

The Autonomous Technologies is a spiral scanning spot with 1 mm beam size. It has a relatively sophisticated tracking system that is only currently being developed by other excimer laser manufacturers (Figure 2-11).

The Novatec Laser Systems is designed for low maintenance cost (Figure 2-12). It is a solid-state laser; unlike all the others, it plugs into the wall. It has an optical zone of up to 10 mm with an automated eye tracking device, and can treat hyperopia and high myopia, as well as regular and irregular

---

Table 2-4.
Flying Spot Approach

- LaserSight Technologies (Compak-200 and LaserScan 2000)
- Autonomous Technologies (T-PRK)
- Novatec Laser Systems (LightBlade$_2$)

Advantages
- Small energy output
- Spot placement can be custom designed
- Easy myopic and hyperopic correction
- Solid-state laser (Novatec Laser Systems) avoids using toxic gases

Disadvantages
- Active tracking system
- Longest operating time
- Clinical data limited to date
- Maintenance of solid-state laser optics unknown (Novatec Laser Systems)

Unique Hardware Features

	LaserSight	**Autonomous**	**Novatec**
Beam Shaping			
Myopia	Scanning spot	Spiral scanning spot	Spiral scanning spot
Astigmatism	Meridional scanning spot	Meridional scanning spot	Linear or elliptical scanning spot
Hyperopia	Annular scanning spot	Annular scanning spot	Annular scanning spot
Beam Smoothing	Scanning alone	Tracking sensor directed scanning	Computer directed scanning
Beam Size	0.8 to 1.2 mm	1 mm	0.01 to 0.5 mm
Beam Energy Density	160 to 300 mJ/cm^2	180 mJ/cm^2	100 mJ/cm^2
Pulse Frequency	100 Hz	100 Hz	>100 Hz
Beam Tracking	None	Active dual axis (Ladar Vision)	Automated, active

Adapted with permission from Talamo JH, Krueger RR, eds. The excimer manual: a clinician's guide to excimer laser surgery. *Boston: Little, Brown and Co; 1997.*

---

astigmatism. It is a scanning machine combined with tracking. The manufacturer states that its tracking system will reduce optical zone decentration.

There are also some non-excimer refracting lasers. These include the intrastromal laser (ISL), which is a neodymium:YAG laser.

Sunrise Technologies (Fremont, California) (Figure 2-13) has developed a holmium laser. This laser, along with the Summit Technology Holmium, is

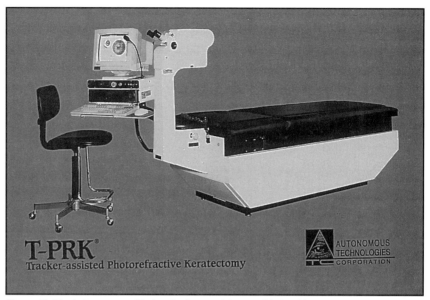

Figure 2-11. Autonomous Technologies spot laser with tracking.

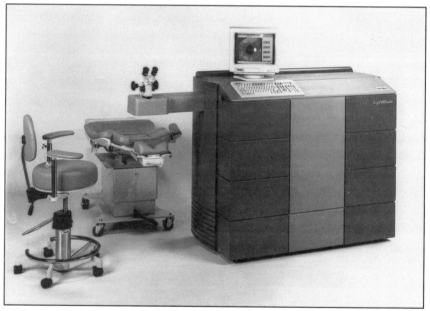

Figure 2-12. Novatec Laser Systems solid-state excimer laser.

used specifically for hyperopic correction.

Marguerite B. McDonald indicated at the time of this writing that Summit Technology has 200 lasers in the United States and 250 in other countries. VisX has 200 lasers placed worldwide (as of May 1, 1996). Undoubtedly, Summit Technology and VisX will proliferate in the United

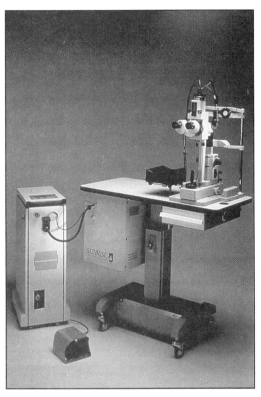

Figure 2-13. Sunrise Technologies holmium: YAG laser.

**Table 2-5.
Current Excimer Lasers Around the World
as of May 1, 1996**

	Summit	VisX	Chiron	Nidek	ATC	Novatec	Aesculap-Meditec	LaserSight
US Units	200	200	19	8	1	9	4	5
Outside US	250	Worldwide	122	123	1	13	200	87
Surface PRK	Yes	Yes	Yes	Yes	Yes	—	—	Yes
LASIK	Yes	Yes	Yes	Yes	Yes	Yes	Yes	Yes
Hyperopic PRK	Yes	Yes	Yes	Yes	Yes	Yes	Yes	No
PARK	Yes	Yes	Yes	Yes	Yes	—	—	No

Courtesy of Marguerite B. McDonald, MD.

States due to their early approval. Other lasers are still in the investigational stages and have not achieved status in the United States for widespread delivery. These are the Photon Data Laser (Winter Park, Florida) and the Telco Laser (Perth, Australia). The numbers of laser units around the world are indicated in Table 2-5.

Patient Eligibility

Population Demographics and Patient Selection

One fifth to one third of all Americans (48 to 79 million people) need eyeglasses or contact lenses to see well at a distance; a majority of older Americans need eyeglasses to read books and to do other fine, close work. Nearly 50% of people between the ages of 18 and 45 are dependent on spectacles or contact lenses to achieve a quality of vision satisfactory for their daily needs.

There are currently about 75 million myopic individuals in North America. Of these, more than 60 million have <6 D of myopia. Myopia is a frequent phenomenon in all social categories, but incidence varies depending on a number of factors (Table 3-1). Data from the 1971 to 1972 National Health and Nutrition Examination Survey were used to estimate myopia prevalence rates for persons in the United States between the ages of 12 and 54 years. Approximately 25% of Americans have myopia, with the right eye commonly being slightly more affected. Whites had substantially higher rates than blacks. For whites and blacks, respectively, rates were 26.3% and 13.0% for right eyes and 25.6% and 12.2% for left eyes.

Myopia has been found to be patterned in its occurrences in different races and ethnic groups. Blacks have been observed to have a low prevalence of myopia. Asians have often been found to have a prevalence of myopia as high as 40%, compared to 20% in whites. Myopia is known to be closely associated in prevalence and severity with educational attainment. It has also been found to be positively associated with social class, degree of urbanization of place of residence, and level of economic development of region or country of residence.

In the National Health and Nutrition Examination Survey, there was little

Table 3-1.
Frequency of Myopia by Social Categories (N=13,536)

Category	% Myopic
Sex	
Male	28.4
Female	35.0
Race	
Black	25.1
Non-black	32.7
Region	
Northeast	32.4
Midwest	35.7
South	24.1
West	33.4
Family Income	
<$500	16.8
$500-$999	20.9
$1,000-$1,999	26.5
$2,000-$2,999	26.7
$3,000-$3,999	28.1
$4,000-$4,999	31.5
$5,000-$6,999	31.2
$7,000-$9,999	32.3
$10,000-$14,999	36.8
≥$15,000	35.1
Grade in School	
≤6th	26.4
7th	28.9
8th	31.3
9th	32.8
10th	32.2
11th	35.4
≥12th	35.0
Age (years)	
12	29.9
13	31.5
14	31.2
15	31.9
16	33.0
17	33.2
Reading Test (deciles)	
1 (low)	19.7
2	24.9
3	27.6
4	30.9
5	31.3
6	32.4
7	31.0
8	38.1
9	37.5
10 (high)	45.3
Time spent reading magazines, books, newspapers in a typical day	
<1 hour	27.7
1-3 hours	32.8
>3 hours	34.6

Source of data: National Health Examination Survey of 12- to 17-year-olds, 1966-1970.

Table 3-2.
Myopia Related to Family Income (Ages 12 to 17)

Family Annual Salary	Incidence of Myopia
<$1,000/year	18%
$1,000-$5,000/year	28%
$5,000-$10,000/year	32%
>$10,000/year	36%

Adapted from Am J Epidemiol. *1980;3:2.*

variation in the overall rates with age. However, there was a progressive increase with age in the proportion of persons with <2 D of myopia and a corresponding decrease in those with ≥2 D of myopia.

The prevalence of myopia increases as average family income rises. For the total population the rates increased from 18% to 28% to 32% to 36% as family income increased (Table 3-2).

Dr. Jack Hartstein has stated that only 3.4% of the population have an astigmatism >3.00 D. This statistic has lulled many ophthalmologists into believing that the other 97% have little or no astigmatism, a statement that is definitely not true. In fact, 34.8% of the population have an astigmatism >1.00 D, and another 24.8% have an astigmatism >1.50 D.

Patient Selection

Most refractive errors are treatable with glasses or contact lenses with small attendant risks (Figure 3-1). Careful patient selection and careful review to the patient of the risk:benefit ratio of excimer laser PRK is a very important consideration.

Patient information and education is a primary prerequisite for PRK. The patient should understand the excimer laser procedure and postoperative evaluation by viewing videotapes, reading printed information sheets, and obtaining information from patient counselors, the surgeon, and other patients.

Eligibility Factors

The following are factors that should be considered:

Age

The patient should be 18 years of age or older. The refraction should be

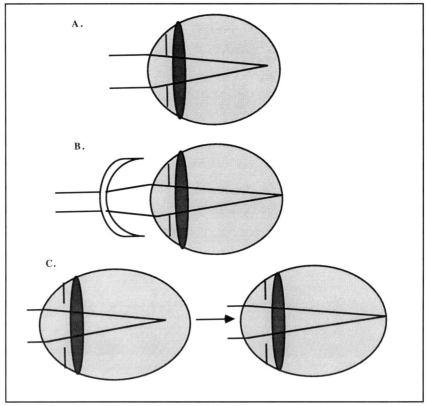

Figure 3-1. (A) An uncorrected myopic eye in which light from the distance comes to a focus in front of the retina. (B) Correction of a myopic eye with a glass or contact lens causes divergence of light rays to create a focus on the retina. (C) Refractive surgery (PRK or RK) can produce flattening of the central cornea resulting in light rays that come to focus on the retina.

relatively stable from the previous year to avoid progressive refractive changes. Some patients between 18 and 21 years of age are interested in a certain level of uncorrected vision to gain employment for occupations such as police work and firefighting. For these patients, refractive stability is not as important.

Presbyopic patients should be instructed that refractive surgery will only correct their distance vision. Patients in their late 30s or early 40s with myopia should be informed that refractive surgery may make it more difficult for them to see at near. They will be trading clarity for distance and losing clarity at near.

Preoperative Evaluation

Knowledge of the previous evaluation is helpful to make certain of

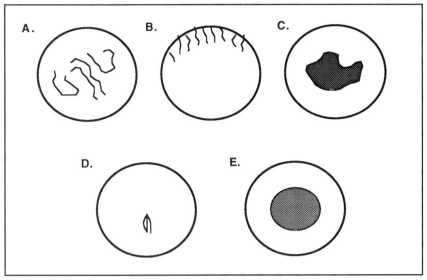

Figure 3-2. Slit lamp examination to detect (A) anterior basement membrane dystrophy, (B) corneal vascularization, (C) corneal scarring, (D) keratoconus, (E) cataract.

stability of the refraction, particularly after discontinuing contact lenses. One should wait to examine the patient for 2 to 3 days after removal of soft contact lenses and 1 month after removal of rigid gas-permeable lenses. Refraction and keratometer readings should be stable on a repeat visit.

Visual Assessment

It is important to measure both uncorrected and best-corrected vision to document for later comparison.

Slit Lamp Examination

The slit lamp examination is used to rule out any significant corneal abnormalities, such as anterior basement membrane dystrophy, vascularization, scarring, or keratoconus, as well as rule out the presence of a cataract (Figure 3-2).

Intraocular Pressure

Since patients are given topical steroids postoperatively, it is important to rule out the presence of glaucoma or a glaucoma suspect who may be more susceptible and vulnerable to raised intraocular pressures (IOPs) with topical steroids.

Fundoscopy

Fundoscopy is a very important exam in myopic patients because there is the possibility of a retinal hole or degenerative retina. It also rules out any optic disc or macular disease as a baseline measurement.

Refraction

The importance of an accurate refraction cannot be overstated. If astigmatism is present, it is extremely important to determine the proper axis. If the cylinder is 15° off axis, the effect from treatment may be decreased by 50%.

Keratometry and Computerized Videokeratography

Although keratometry can be useful, computerized videokeratography, which has become the standard of care, is done prior to laser surgery to rule out subtle abnormalities of the cornea.

True keratoconus is a relative contraindication to laser surgery. There are a variety of diagnostic signs to rule out this disease, including Munson's sign, apical scarring, Vogt's striae, distorted keratometric mires, Placido disk abnormality, and abnormal retinoscopy reflex. However, with videokeratography it is possible to identify early keratoconus or "keratoconus suspect," corneal warpage, and asymmetric or irregular astigmatism (Figure 3-3). Each condition has a different prognosis.

Patients with keratoconus often have irregular astigmatism, and the laser currently is not capable of correcting this abnormality. Hence, if laser surgery were performed to correct the myopia, rigid contact lenses would be required to correct the irregular astigmatism. Nevertheless, there are still uncertainties with respect to keratoconus and the excimer.

Pupil Size

One should refrain from operating on individuals with very large pupils (>6 mm) without at least forewarning them about the possible effects on night driving and glare. As optical zones and transition zones become larger, this complication will be less common.

Avocation and Vocation

The patient's occupation and hobbies have to be considered when planning the surgery because postoperative vision is often diminished in the early stages, although it should gradually improve over days to weeks. The patient should understand the possibility of haze and glare, which are most significant at 2 to 4 months and gradually resolve over time.

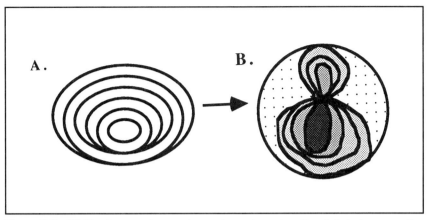

Figure 3-3. (A) Keratoscope image shows rings closer together inferiorly suggestive of keratoconus. (B) Videokeratography represents the computer-generated dioptric map derived from the keratoscope image. In keratoconus, the steeper area is highlighted by a warmer color inferiorly.

Patient Reasons for Undergoing Excimer Laser Surgery

In reviewing our patients' reasons for undergoing PRK, 65% simply wanted to be free of glasses or contact lenses, 25% were contact lens intolerant, 6% chose PRK for sports reasons, and 4% for occupational or professional reasons.

The majority of patients that become contact lens intolerant have dry eyes. Other problems associated with contact lens complications include giant papillary conjunctivitis, hypersensitivity reactions to contact lens solutions, and corneal infiltrates or ulcers.

The excimer laser has great value for patients who are active in a variety of sports, such as swimming, racquet sports, and contact sports. In a variety of professions, a certain level of uncorrected acuity is required for acceptance. As a consequence, there is a significant interest from patients seeking employment in the police force, firefighting, railway lines, and piloting.

Contraindications

Certain criteria should be kept in mind to avoid possible postoperative complications.

Refraction Anomalies

Patients with progressive myopia should be excluded until stabilization of the refraction. Progressive myopia might indicate pathologic myopia. Abnormal corneal topography is an important consideration because a keratoconus suspect might have less than satisfactory results after PRK. A fluctuating refractive error may also indicate diabetes, which should be excluded and controlled.

Ocular Pathologies

Certain types of corneal disorders (eg, keratoconus, pellucid marginal degeneration), advanced keratitis sicca with superficial punctate keratopathy or corneal filaments, and diffuse vascularization are contraindications for PRK. Other contraindications for the excimer laser procedure include uveitis, cataract, retinopathies, and lagophthalmos.

Systemic Pathologies

Patients with active systemic connective tissue diseases (eg, systemic lupus, rheumatoid arthritis) are considered poor PRK candidates because of the potential for poor epithelial healing and the risk of a corneal melt.

Summary

Careful attention must be given to patient selection and preoperative evaluation to maximize the visual results from the PRK procedure. Otherwise, one may be faced with a disappointed patient.

Chapter 4

Benefits of Excimer Laser Treatment

Since the late 1970s, more than 1 1/2 million refractive surgeries have been performed, the majority of those being radial keratotomy (RK). Advances in technology and development of the excimer laser have made refractive surgery highly predictable, with the vast majority of patients having their vision corrected to 20/40 or better with a single treatment. Today, thousands of patients in the world with refractive errors are benefiting from PRK.

Surgery with the excimer laser is more reproducible than a hand-held surgical knife. A laser excision occurs without any deformation of the target tissues. The absence of corneal deformation should permit real-time monitoring of the induced change in the corneal curvature.

Motivations for Excimer Surgery

"Glasses free" and "contact lens free" are top priorities for a great majority of patients with refractive errors because they have been dependent on spectacles or contact lenses. These lenses may impose restrictions on the activities of their lifestyle.

There are many factors that motivate patients to desire surgery. In reviewing our patients' reasons for laser treatment, we found the following categories were mentioned most.

Independence from Optical Devices

The reasons given at our institute for independence from optical devices are (Table 4-1):

1. Cosmetic (65%). There are very important positive psychological effects of being spectacle free. These patients wish to see well at all times with-

Table 4-1. Reasons for Seeking Refractive Surgery	
250 Consecutive Cases from the Bochner Eye Institute	
Cosmetic	65%
Contact Lens Intolerance	25%
Sports	6%
Professional/Occupational	4%

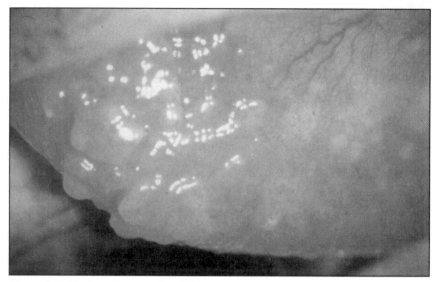

Figure 4-1. Giant papillary conjunctivitis.

out having to wear glasses or contact lenses.

2. Contact lens intolerance (25%). The majority of patients who become contact lens intolerant have dry eyes. Other problems associated with contact lens complications include giant papillary conjunctivitis (Figure 4-1), hypersensitivity reactions to contact lens solutions, and corneal infiltrates or ulcers (Figure 4-2). Some patients are also unable to handle the daily problems of insertion and removal of contact lenses. These patients welcome laser treatment.

3. Sports (6%). Both glasses and contacts can pose restrictions to playing baseball, football, hockey, basketball, racquet sports (Figure 4-3), contact sports, and swimming, among others.

4. Professional or occupational reasons (4%).

Occupational Reasons

Frequently, the need to use glasses or contact lenses is an important

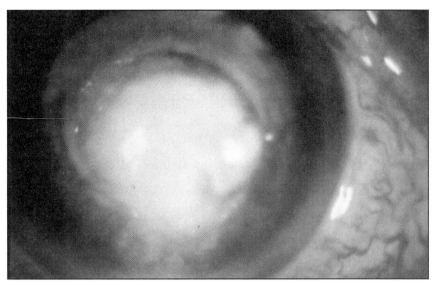

Figure 4-2. Corneal ulcer in a contact lens wearer secondary to pseudomonas.

restriction to certain types of employment, because in a variety of professions, a certain level of uncorrected acuity is required for acceptance. These workers include pilots, police officers, firefighters, railway workers, cooks (glasses fog up with steam), and airline flight attendants (contact lenses and spectacles are frequently disallowed by some airlines for safety reasons).

Following Other Surgeries

One of the clinical indications for excimer laser surgery is the correction of refractive errors following other ocular surgery (Figure 4-4). The excimer laser can refine the visual outcome.

After RK Surgery

The excimer laser appears to be an effective treatment for patients who remain undercorrected after RK. While undercorrection can be managed with spectacles or contact lenses, most patients have RK done because they don't want to wear glasses or contact lenses. Secondary procedures are common among RK recipients. The excimer can save a failed RK result after repeat RK procedures. The results, however, are not as good as a primary excimer laser ablation.

After Penetrating Keratoplasty

Excimer laser can be used to treat anisometropia after corneal transplantation. Many patients may be disappointed in their surgery despite

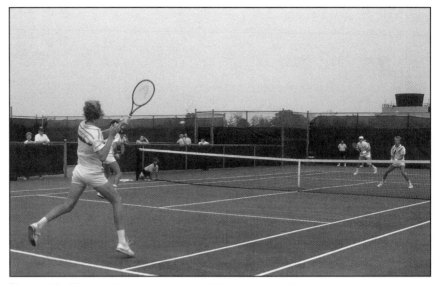

Figure 4-3. Glasses often impose a restriction in competitive racquet sports such as tennis.

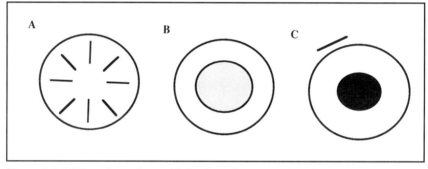

Figure 4-4. PRK can be performed following other types of surgical procedures to correct myopia and/or astigmatism: (A) RK, (B) corneal transplantation, (C) cataract surgery.

clear transplants with 20/20 corrected vision because of induced myopia or astigmatism. Safety is a concern in these patients, but in our practice we have found no significant corneal haze or increased risk of graft rejection after laser treatment.

After Cataract Surgery

Intraocular lenses (IOLs) were developed for cataract surgery patients to eliminate the need to wear contact lenses or spectacles. However, surgery may induce myopia and/or astigmatism. Excimer laser treatment seems a good alternative to minimize these post-cataract refractive problems.

Summary

Patients seek out refractive surgery for a variety of reasons. The majority of refractive surgery conducted in the United States has been RK. The excimer laser is a more predictable and efficacious alternative. It is noteworthy that in our practice 95% of patients undergoing PRK request their second eye be operated upon with the excimer laser, which attests to the success of treatment to the first eye.

Chapter 5

Psychological Support

Psychosocial factors can influence the patient's decision-making and treatment evaluation processes. It is essential that patients understand the preoperative evaluation and necessary tests, all steps of the excimer laser procedure itself, and postoperative evaluations. In addition to talking with the surgeon and patient counselor or liaison, patients can also obtain important information through videotapes, patient brochures, information sheets, or patients who have undergone the PRK procedure. Good communication between the surgeon and patient establishes trust. A trained patient counselor or physician who has had the PRK procedure is a very positive psychological boost for the patient.

Preoperative Discussions

The decision to have surgery is a "partnership" decision between the patient and physician. If the eyes are "normal" and correctable to 20/20, then PRK is elective surgery to suit the patient's schedule.

The aim of this surgery is to improve the quality of life of the patient. For this reason, total and open discussion with the patient of pros and cons and what to expect and what not to expect are very important.

Never promise that the patient will be "glasses free." This creates a mindset that can quickly turn to hostility if glasses are subsequently required.

The presbyopic myope should know that with complete visual correction reading glasses will be required. The patient is trading distance for reading glasses and can then make an informed decision whether or not to have the surgery.

Tell the patient the stated statistics, if possible, of the percent of visual improvement. With up to 6 D of myopia, there is a 96% chance of obtaining 20/40 or better uncorrected vision within 2 to 4 weeks. These types of statistics are important to bring freedom from worry.

Most of these patients will know very little about surgical treatment. Talk the patient through the PRK procedure, explaining what to expect during and after the procedure. Excimer laser patients may also need information about pain, medications, activity restrictions, possible complications and symptoms, treatments, postoperative vision, length of stay, and plans for follow-up care.

Operative Discussions

Patients have different perceptions of their situation and different levels of stress or anxiety. The surgeon must talk to the patient and explain what is happening during surgery. This discussion should include descriptions of what the patient might feel, see, smell, or hear during his or her surgical procedure. It also gives the patient information about the sequence of these events. Sensory information can lessen the stress or discomfort associated with excimer laser surgery. Communication between the ophthalmologist and patient is very important because the patient needs to maintain fixation and remain motionless for a finite period of time.

At the conclusion of the procedure, demonstrate to patients that they can see better, which gives patients a tremendous positive psychological boost. Patients may choose to discard their old glasses, which can be used for indigent patients in third world countries.

Postoperative Discussions

Excimer patients should expect vision to get blurry while the epithelium is healing. They should know that symptoms such as ghosting, glare, and shadows are transient phenomena and will disappear.

The practitioner must spend a good portion of postoperative visits talking to the patient and explaining what is happening. One must instruct the patient about hygiene and the increased risk of infection during the first few days while the epithelium is healing.

Changing Acuity After Excimer Laser Treatment

Changes in vision with healing of epithelium and stroma is normal during the early postoperative course. For this reason the eye practitioner has to spend time with patients to discuss their progress and be available to answer their questions and concerns.

Regression of a good achieved result may occur and the patient may regain some of his or her refractive error. Careful titration of the steroid or nonsteroidal drugs may be required in order to modulate the result and prevent slippage. If there is slippage of the refractive error, emphasize that a "touch-up" can subsequently be done with the excimer laser to bring back restored visual acuity.

Effect on Work, Hobbies, Vacations, and Trips

The vision could have a delay in recovery especially after having bilateral PRK surgery. There could be a problem in working shortly thereafter, or interference with hobbies, vacation, or travel.

A patient should always allow more than enough time for healing to occur before resumption of activities requiring critical vision.

Realistic Refractive Outcomes Expectations

The patient should have realistic refractive outcomes expectations. The ideal outcome would be one in which the patient can see very soon afterwards, at least as well without glasses or contact lens as he or she had previously been able to see with the best possible glasses or contacts, and do so with no side effects. In reality, however, the outcome is usually something less than this in one or more respects and is sometimes considerably less. It is very important that the patient's expectations are reasonable and that he or she understands the possible ways in which his or her expectations might not be met.

Pregnancy and Refractive Surgery

When a woman is pregnant or nursing, there may be hormonal changes that could affect the measurement of myopia, hyperopia, or astigmatism. As well, medications (sedation, pain medications, and even eyedrops) can be transmitted to the fetus by the mother's bloodstream or to the baby through breast milk. For these reasons, refractive surgery should not be performed on a pregnant woman or a nursing mother.

Flying or Scuba Diving Following Surgery

Patients are often concerned about pressure changes with flying or scuba diving after PRK surgery. These pressure changes will not affect the healing or outcome of the surgery. It is safe to fly anytime after PRK surgery or scuba dive as early as 1 week after surgery.

Corneal Topography

Chapter 6

Videokeratography

omputerized videokeratography is used in the pre- and postoperative assessments of PRK patients. Preoperatively, the topography maps are used mainly to rule out keratoconus but also are valuable in detecting corneal warpage from contact lenses and other pathologies. Postoperatively, computerized videokeratoscopy is useful in diagnosing decentered ablations, central islands, or asymmetrical astigmatism. Postoperatively, the maps may show changes in steepening in the ablation zone prior to the development of clinical regression. A postoperative map is essential in order to obtain a difference map postoperatively.

Computerized corneal topographic analysis is the measurement of the curvature of the anterior corneal surface. This tool is based on the principles of keratometry and photokeratoscopy developed in 1880 by Placido (Figure 6-1). He placed a planar target with concentric alternating black and white rings in front of a patient's eye and then observed the shape of the rings in the virtual image of that target created from the reflection off of the patient's anterior corneal surface (Figure 6-2). If the cornea is spherical, the rings appear circular and concentric. Deviations of the corneal shape appear as either distortions in shape or eccentricity of the rings (Figure 6-3).

Photokeratoscopy provides the user with only qualitative information about the curvature of the cornea, changes that accompany surgery, and progressive corneal abnormalities. The keratometer yields quantitative data, but only at four points. These points are located at approximately the 3-mm optical zone along two perpendicular meridians. One pair of points is aligned along the steepest axis of the corneal surface, with the second pair

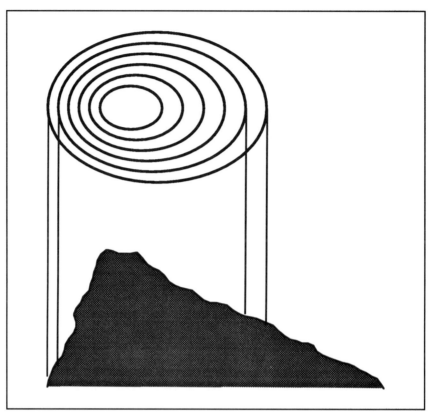

Figure 6-1. Photokeratoscopy is similar to aerial topography maps showing areas that are relatively flat or steep.

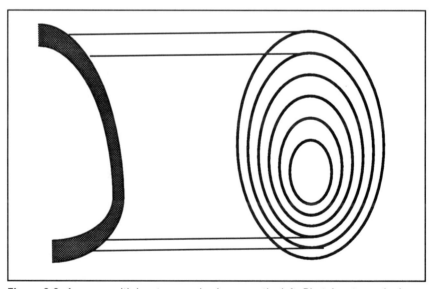

Figure 6-2. A cornea with keratoconus is shown on the left. Photokeratograph shown on the right with evidence of inferior steepening as noted by the rings being closer together.

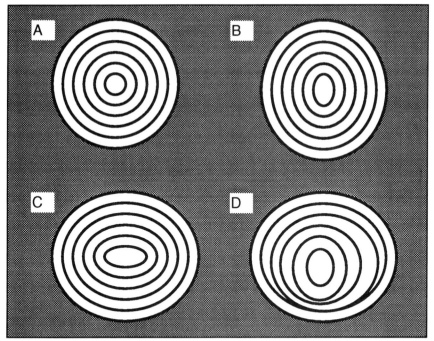

Figure 6-3. Photokeratoscopy images showing (A) spherical cornea, (B) against-the-rule astigmatism, (C) with-the-rule astigmatism, (D) keratoconus.

90° away. Each pair of points is averaged across its respective meridian to yield two K values, which approximate the cornea's central refractive power. The keratometer has fundamental limitations in that it is able only to measure points along the annulus of the 3-mm optical zone, and it assumes orthogonal symmetry of the flat and steep axis of the cornea (Figure 6-4).

With the capabilities of modern computers and software technology to qualify the data obtained from reflected Placido disk images, it has become feasible and practical to precisely analyze the radius of curvature (mm) and corresponding refractive power (D) at 6000 to 8000 points on the corneal surface from inside the 1-mm optical zone to outside the 9-mm optical zone. This information is then translated into a complete color-coded representation of the cornea's shape. These topographic maps provide the ability to monitor corneal curvature changes from the apex to the periphery.

There are a variety of Placido disk based systems available: EyeSys, Tomey, Alcon EyeMap, Humphrey, etc. All the systems have advantages and disadvantages. Variables include the number of data points measured, the working distance for focusing, automated or manual focusing, sensitivity to the central vs. peripheral cornea, and nomograms for interpretation. The EyeSys Corneal Analysis System uses a back-lit conical

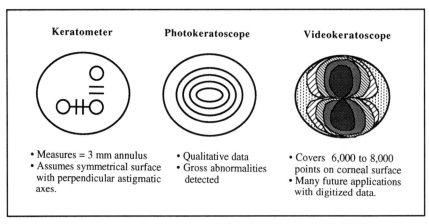

Figure 6-4. Comparison of the keratometer, photokeratoscope, and videokeratoscope.

dish as its Placido target (Figure 6-5); other systems use a cylindrical light cone as the Placido target. With either a conical dish or a cylindrical light cone, a Placido ring image is produced on the cornea. With today's instruments, the videocamera (the observer) visualizes the virtual image of the black and white Placido ring pattern on the eye. The computer then analyzes this digitized video image and displays the data in a variety of useful formats.

Non-Placido disk based systems include the PAR and Orbscan. The PAR system projects a grid onto the cornea and measures the reflected image after fluorescein has been instilled in the tear film. A shape or elevation map can be determined in addition to measuring corneal curvature. The Orbscan takes multiple cross-sectional scans of the cornea and is able to determine the shape of both the anterior and posterior cornea and pachymetry values.

For Figures 6-5 through 6-12, see the Color Insert between pages 74 and 75.

Corneal Topography Analysis in PRK

The development and evaluation of keratorefractive surgery have benefited from the parallel advances made in the field of corneal topography analysis.

A major advantage of PRK is the precision with which the excimer laser ablates corneal tissue. Consistent, accurate centration of the procedure is one component of the technique that is critical to its success.

From the topographic map of a cornea, it is possible to determine the amount of spherocylindrical aberration before surgery and objective measurement of surgical results, as well as the precise location of the ablation zone in photorefractive surgery.

Preoperative Analysis

The normal cornea is aspheric, being steepest centrally with progressive flattening toward the periphery. One form of commonly encountered corneal topographic finding is that of regular and symmetric astigmatism with a bow-tie shape. A with-the-rule regular corneal cylinder is vertically aligned, while against-the-rule corneal astigmatism takes the form of a horizontally aligned bow-tie pattern.

The steepest axis of the cornea may not be symmetric. Asymmetrically distributed astigmatism has potentially important implications in surgical correction. For patients who have asymmetric astigmatism, it is very important to ask about contact lens wear, and whether there is a family history of keratoconus.

Although topography is important in achieving good visual outcomes, it is essential to ensure that the cornea is stable prior to performing any refractive procedure. Operating on an unstable cornea usually leads to disappointing visual outcomes.

Corneal warpage is a change in the contour of the cornea with resultant change in refraction. This condition is not as prevalent today with rigid gas-permeable lenses as it was in the era of polymethyl methacrylate (PMMA) lenses. It is important to distinguish between corneal warpage induced by contact lenses and true keratoconus. Since differentiation may be difficult, the patient must abstain from wearing contact lenses until refraction and corneal topography are stable. Significant changes suggest that corneal warpage from contact lenses has not yet resolved. If contact lens wear is discontinued only a few days prior to the preoperative evaluation, the final refractive result may be unsuitable because the time for re-establishment of corneal stability after contact lens warpage may take hours to months to occur. Stability can vary with soft lenses from minutes to 1 week or longer. One month is the minimum for discontinuation of rigid gas-permeable lenses, although it may take 6 months or longer before the cornea is stable. On a practical note, if serial refractions performed every 2 weeks show no change in refraction (<0.50 D) and computerized videokeratography is stable and appears normal, it is probably safe to proceed with laser surgery.

The preoperative identification of early or mild keratoconus is very important because refractive surgery is generally not beneficial to these patients. Any irregular astigmatism cannot be satisfactorily treated with the excimer laser. Even if the myopia were reduced, any residual irregular astigmatism would require a rigid contact lens for correction. In addition, the correction of asymmetric astigmatism is difficult to treat with the present laser machines as more laser pulses would be required at the steeper quadrant compared to the meridian 180° away. The other concern of treating unrecognized keratoconus patients is the potential for litigation if keratoconus is detected postoperatively and is thought to be caused by the laser procedure.

Obviously, patients with advanced keratoconus, showing Vogt's striae, do not require computerized videokeratography to make the diagnosis. It is the patient who presents with a clear cornea and less than 20/20 visual acuity who needs corneal topography.

The keratometer is helpful if corneal mires are irregular or distorted, and the cornea is relatively steep. However, if the cornea is relatively flat, then the diagnosis may be keratoconus, anterior basement dystrophy, or a tear film abnormality.

For these patients, computerized topography is valuable. The Holladay map, used by the EyeSys system, provides an estimate of the potential acuity at different areas on the cornea. The most crucial area for PRK patients is the central 6 mm of the cornea. In fact, patients with inferior steepening on Placido disk exams who have excellent best-corrected visual acuity and a relatively normal Holladay map may actually have a cornea that is a variation of normal and not early keratoconus.

The PAR maps are also useful in these cases because they show true elevation and depression; this quality may help differentiate a normal cornea from one with keratoconus. The shape map may show that the inferior cornea is bulging anteriorly consistent with keratoconus. If the curvature map shows inferior steepening, but the shape map shows only that the apex of the cornea has been displaced inferiorly without the inferior cornea bulging forward, this condition may be a variation of normal. Longitudinal studies are required to determine if a percentage of these patients develop clinical keratoconus.

The Orbscan topography system, while still early in its development, also provides true elevation and depression maps, as well as a map of pachymetry values that describe corneal thickness measurements distributed across the cornea. When the apex has been displaced inferiorly and is associated with the most prominent area of thinning, the surgeon can be confident of a keratoconus diagnosis.

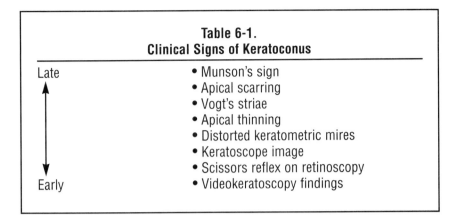

Table 6-1. Clinical Signs of Keratoconus	
Late ↑ ↓ Early	• Munson's sign • Apical scarring • Vogt's striae • Apical thinning • Distorted keratometric mires • Keratoscope image • Scissors reflex on retinoscopy • Videokeratoscopy findings

Corneal topography of family members of patients with keratoconus often demonstrates that some members appear to be affected by mild forms of the disease without overt clinical signs such as apical protrusion and thinning, epithelial iron line, Vogt's striae, and retinoscopic or keratometry abnormalities.

There are a variety of clinical signs of keratoconus that can be used to make the diagnosis (Table 6-1). The most subtle abnormalities are detected with corneal topography (Figures 6-6 and 6-7). Criteria were hypothesized by Rabinowitz to identify patients with keratoconus:

- Central corneal power >46.5 D
- Asymmetry in central corneal power between the two eyes >0.92 D
- Greater steepening inferior, I-S value >1.6 D

Videokeratoscopy manufacturers are trying to incorporate these data into software programs that will provide statistics on the probability that a patient has keratoconus. Based on our findings and the literature, we suggest corneal topography be used to screen all patients prior to PRK.

Topography is helpful in predicting outcomes. For example, patients achieve better visual results if their refractive astigmatic axes approximate their topographic axes. Theoretically, in these cases, PRK that treats astigmatism can create a spherical cornea. These patients, especially low to moderate myopes, may achieve outstanding acuity levels due to the creation of a spherical cornea.

Surgeons, if they have access to more than one topography unit, need to remember that different machines measure differently. That means the astigmatic axis can vary from machine to machine by 1° to 20° due to soft- and hardware variables.

Analysis of the Centration of PRK

Accurate centration PRK is one component of the technique that is critical to its success (Figures 6-8 and 6-9). Objective measurement of corneal surface topography is an important tool in determining centration of PRK.

PRK decentration relative to the entrance pupil may produce increased glare and distortion from the edge of the ablation zone encountering the edge of the pupil (see Figure 6-9). Eccentric ablation zones always result in manifest refractive astigmatism.

The keratography is processed using the pupil-finding software. The pupillary center is indicated by a dot. The center of the post-PRK flat zone is estimated visually in the differential map by subtracting the preoperative keratography from the postoperative keratography. The flat zone is generally a confluent central circle of blue hues. The computer cursor "+" sign is moved to that location. The distance from the center of the ablation zone to the pupillary center is recorded directly from the legend in both millimeters and meridian degrees.

Decentration of the ablation zone can cause an increase in corneal astigmatism measurable by videokeratography. Eyes with higher attempted correction have a greater probability of decentration of the ablated zone because these patients have greater difficulty in maintaining fixation during treatment, due either to their greater myopia or to the longer time required for laser treatment.

Evaluating centration of the PRK by visually comparing the keratography obtained before and after treatment can give a false sense of the ablation zone (Figure 6-10). The differential map, which is a point for point subtraction of the preoperative map from the postoperative map, is essential to correctly analyze the centration of PRK. In some cases, the post-PRK map may appear to show a marked decentration, but the difference map may indicate a well-centered ablation (Figure 6-11). The appearance of decentration on the postoperative map is due to preexisting asymmetric astigmatism.

Postoperative topography is helpful in assessing both symptomatic and asymptomatic patients. It provides feedback to the surgeon on the centration of the ablation. Patients with small pupils may be asymptomatic yet still have a slight or moderate decentration.

Halos experienced postoperatively may be caused by epithelial irregularity, a pupil that is larger than the ablative zone, or a decentered ablation. Computerized videokeratography allows one to rule out halos secondary to a decentered ablation. Epithelial irregularity generally resolves within a few months, leaving a smooth transition from the normal epithelium to the epithelium over the ablated area. Halos caused by a pupil that is larger than the ablation zone size are difficult to correct. This situation should have been assessed preoperatively. Patients can be retreated with excimer lasers with larger optical zones.

The cornea's healing response post-PRK can create the impression that the ablation was decentered. To obtain an accurate assessment of the surgeon's skill in centering the procedure over the pupil, a difference map should be obtained 1 month postoperatively. We have seen difference maps at 1 month showing perfect centration and at periods after this that appear decentered. Thickening of the epithelium or the laying down of new collagen are probably responsible for these topographic changes.

Central Islands

The ideal contour of a cornea after PRK would be a homogeneously flat central zone, but many investigators have noted in some patients an increase in the central power (central bump or central island) on topography maps (Figure 6-12). The etiology of these bumps or islands is not clear. A number of theories have been proposed:

- Plume theory, in which the vaporized molecules interfere with the laser beam centrally
- Optical degradation
- Shockwave theory, in which fluid from the cornea is pushed centrally during the procedure and interferes with the laser beam
- Epithelial hyperplasia, in which the regrowth of epithelium results in thickening or hyperplasia to the central cornea

The islands usually measure <2.5 mm in size and are over 1 D in height. In the majority of cases, the islands resolve spontaneously over a period of weeks to months. Chronic central islands (>6 months) that are visually significant can be treated with the excimer laser. True central islands are relatively easy to treat. Paracentral islands are more difficult to treat since the exact location is not in the center of the pupil.

Placido disk based systems generally measure curvature and not shape. Therefore, the differentiation of a central elevation from a divot may be difficult. A central island may, in fact, be a central divot created by too deep a prophylactic central island treatment. The worst possible management of a divot is to perform additional laser treatment. In these eyes, the Placido disk technology will show a similar map between an island and a divot. The PAR and Orbscan systems occasionally show depressed central areas that appear as true islands with Placido disk systems. Further refinements in the accuracy of all these topography machines will enable us to clearly differentiate a central island from a divot. If at all possible it is best to wait for these focal areas of steepening to resolve spontaneously.

Summary

Computerized videokeratography is an important tool for the refractive surgeon. In our practice, it is an integral part of the preoperative evaluation and the postoperative period. The slit lamp is not of great clinical value in assessing patients who complain of postoperative halos, glare, or monocular diplopia. Computerized topography, however, often enables the clinician to make the correct diagnosis. Its value postoperatively is not only to evaluate subjective complaints, but to give feedback to the surgeon on his or her centration technique. In the future, these instruments may be used to directly input data into the laser computer so that laser pulses can be distributed to produce a more spherical cornea.

Technique

Technical Operation of the Excimer Laser

The term *excited dimer* refers to any diatomic molecule in which the component atoms are bound in the excited state but are not bound in the ground state. Excimer lasers are pulsed gas lasers that use a mixture of a rare gas and a halogen as the active medium to create an excited dimer.

Laser Construction

The most important part of an excimer laser is the lasing cavity that consists of the gas reservoir, input system for high-voltage electricity, and mirrors. One end of the lasing cavity has holes to allow the passage of only coherent radiation. This end is connected to the IBM computer-controlled, translating slit delivery system, which consists of a complex system of mirrors, lenses, and prisms (Figure 7-1).

In the delivery system, the laser beam is expanded by a lens and diverted toward the eye through a series of mirrors. It passes through the calibrated slit mask, and the image of the slit is passed through a rotating dove prism that can change the orientation of the slit under computer control. The objective lens moves in the x, y, and z directions under computer control and moves the slit image over the surface of the cornea.

Operation

As there are many excimer lasers available (see Table 2-1) we will confine our remarks to the lasers with which we have the greatest experience: the VisX 20/20 B and STAR, broad beam lasers, and the Nidek

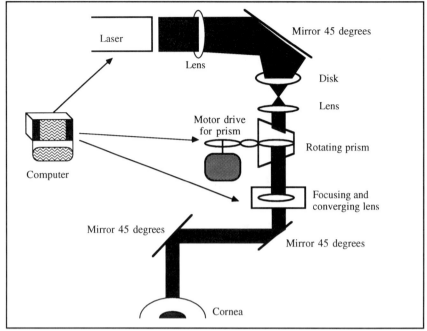

Figure 7-1. Example of excimer laser delivery system. Modified from Hanna KD, Chastan JC, Asfar L, et al. *J Cataract Refract Surg.* 1989;15:390-396.

EC-5000 laser, a scanning laser.

The VisX Lasers

The VisX 20/20 B and STAR lasers use a fluence of 160 mJ/cm^2 and a repetition rate of 6 Hz. These models will serve as examples of the state-of-the-art in broad beam excimer laser technology.

Before the system is used, the gas status should be checked (Figure 7-2). The user should verify that the hose on the liquid nitrogen tank is mounted to the "liquid" port, not the "vent" port, and then turn on the tank. The next step is to verify the tank level on the tank gauge (full, 1/2, 1/4, <1/4). The valve with the blue handle on the gas panel of the premix tank should be open and the tank on. The tank pressure should be >100 psi. The valves on the nitrogen and halogen tanks should be open, and the pressure of both tanks should be >500 psi.

The system can then be turned on. The computer control station and energy meter should both be on. The suction should be operative, as well as the patient fixation light. On the VisX 20/20 B, the green light on the cryo gas purifier (API) should also be on. Finally, the functions of the patient chair should be verified.

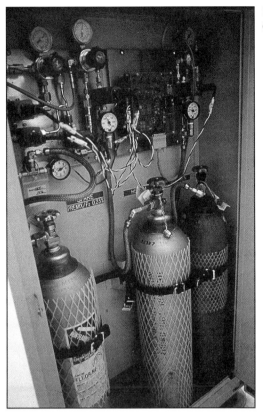

Figure 7-2. Laser gases in rear of excimer laser.

Safety Checks

The calibration of the excimer laser is of utmost importance in achieving excellent visual results. The first safety check is to ablate a PMMA test block with the phototherapeutic keratectomy (PTK) mode and view the plastic under the lensometer (Figures 7-3 through 7-5). The test block should read 0 D if the surface is smooth. If a plus reading is obtained, then there may be decreased laser pulses to the center of the plastic caused by degradation of the optics. If the plastic is satisfactory, then one moves on to performing a test in PRK mode.

In PRK mode we usually ablate a -4.00 D at 6 mm. The test block should read -4.00 D on the lensometer. The reading can be blurry due to ablation pattern. If the reading is -3.50 D, then the depth per pulse is decreased (which increases the number of pulses) and the test block is again ablated. If the reading is -4.50 D, then the depth per pulse is increased (which decreases the number of pulses) and the test block is ablated again. If the test block reads -4.00 D at a given depth per pulse, then the system is properly calibrated.

It is important to grossly evaluate the ablation with a magnifying lens so

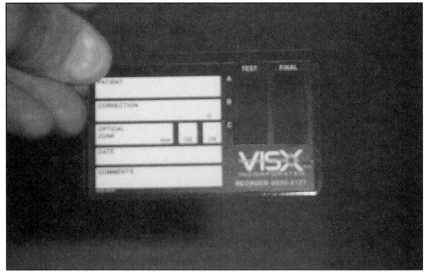

Figure 7-3. Plastic used to measure fluence and quality of ablation surface and size.

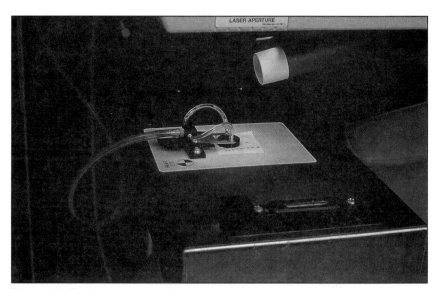

Figure 7-4. Testing plate for centration check.

as to view the concentric rings, to be assured that there are no pits or protrusions on the surface and that the size is exactly what has been programmed into the computer (Figure 7-6). The shape of rings must be circular. If the shape is elliptical, the dove prism of axis, or plastic slide, is not horizontal.

The plastic disc (test block) may be sent to a laboratory to be measured on the Datatech (special micrometer test gauge) instrument, which can accurately evaluate the effect on the test block and determine whether the

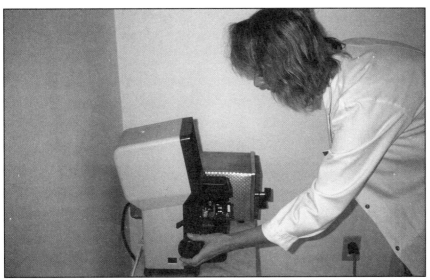

Figure 7-5. Measurement of refractive change with lensometer.

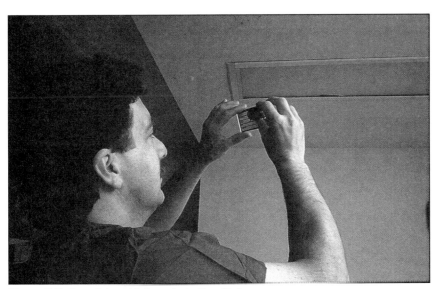

Figure 7-6. Examining ablation of plastic with loupe.

beam is homogeneous and of good quality (Figures 7-7A and 7-7B).

One of the most important safety checks is to be sure that the laser beam is centered properly underneath the microscope. With the VisX 20/20 B, a piece of paper is ablated and the discoloration of the paper observed through the microscope to make sure that the left reticule is directly aligned with the ablation zone. With the STAR laser, a test block of plastic is ablated, which should be centerd within the projected red reticule. If the laser beam is not well aligned, an adjustment is made and a reablation is performed.

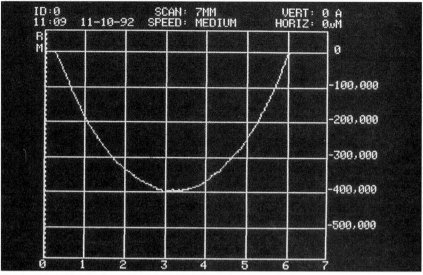

Figure 7-7A. Datatech testing of plastic. Good ablation pattern.

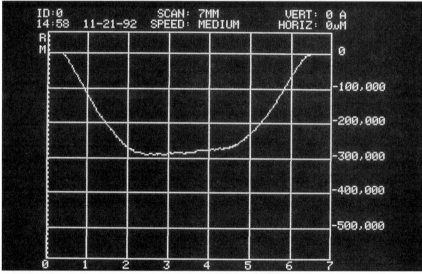

Figure 7-7B. Abnormal pattern with diminished central depth.

Features of the VisX STAR

- Projected binocular red reticule for easy centration over the patient pupil
- No nitrogen gas required
- Small ceramic gas cavity which decreases gas utilization
- Fan that circulates air around optics to keep them cleaner and hence decreases the replacement rate

- Joystick for accurate centration and focusing with x, y, and z control
- User-friendly computer interface
- Direct and indirect illumination that allows improved visibility
- Myopic, astigmatic, and hyperopic modules

The broad beam STAR laser has a maximum optical zone of 6 mm for myopia and astigmatism. The use of multipass and multizone techniques results in a smoother ablation. The laser works in a scanning mode to create a 9-mm hyperopic ablation.

The Nidek EC-5000 Laser

Nidek (Tokyo, Japan) began development in 1985 with Drs. Carmen Puliafito and Roger Steinert. Nidek commenced production in 1992.

Nidek has an ablation rate calibration mode for PRK and hyperopia. The calibration for PRK is preprogrammed for -3.00 D at 5 mm with a laser pulse repetition rate of 40 Hz and desired ablation rate on plate of 0.3 μm/scan. The above calibration is sufficient when the intention is to treat ≤7.5 mm zones. If treatment at zones >7.5 mm is required, a second calibration is done at expanded area calibration which is -2.00 D at 5-mm zone with laser pulse repetition rate of 40 Hz and desired ablation rate on plate of 0.2 μm/scan.

The PMMA test block should read -3.00 D for normal area calibration and -2.00 D for expanded area calibration. Findings of the lensometer are entered into the computer. The computer will advise for repeat calibration or self-adjustment.

Because the hyperopic transition zone is >7.5 mm, the above calibrations are required for hyperopic correction. Hyperopic calibration must be done before every single procedure unless the hyperopic corrections are the same.

The objective correction diopter in hyperopic calibration mode is half the correction value on the patient eye with a treatment zone of 5.5 mm and a transition zone of 9.0 mm. The reading by lensometer is entered into the computer. The difference should be under 10%. The accuracy of the operations directly depends on this result.

It is important to grossly evaluate the ablation with a magnifying lens so as to view the concentric rings (same as with VisX). The laser beam is fixed and centered underneath the microscope. The reticule is directly aligned with the ablation zone.

Features of the Nidek EC-5000

- Smooth and uniform ablated surface due to scanning mechanism

- Low temperature elevation because of the scanning feature on the cornea
- Transition zone: ablated and non-ablated surface are connected smoothly
- Alignment: controlled by three-dimensional motorized joystick

The Nidek laser has a maximum optical zone of 6.5 mm for myopia and astigmatism and transition zone of 7.5 mm. For hyperopia, its optical zone is 5.5 mm and transition zone up to 9.0 mm.

It is said that the scanning property of the Nidek leaves a more uniform surface. It is low on gas costs and optics degradation due to a constant flow of nitrogen gas through the optics. Premixed gas can be used for up to 20 refills per cylinder and helium for 50 refills per cylinder.

The newest software also contains a cylinder correction compensation for myopic astigmatism and astigmatic prescription. Also, the amount of overcorrection after only astigmatic prescriptions is calculated automatically; a plano -3.00 D will not only need to be corrected for 3 D astigmatism, but also for approximately +1.00 D overcorrection in hyperopic mode.

Chapter 8

Surgical Technique

The excimer laser is used to vaporize a precise amount of corneal tissue in a preprogrammed manner to alter the curvature of the cornea and reduce or eliminate myopia, hyperopia, and/or astigmatism. This procedure has been named photorefractive keratectomy, or PRK. To remove anterior corneal tissue to remove opacities and other corneal disease, the procedure is called phototherapeutic keratectomy, or PTK.

The PRK surgical technique consists of ablating a lens-shaped volume of tissue from the stroma. The shape or contour of the ablated area in the treatment of myopia is achieved by allowing more laser energy to strike the central than the peripheral portion of the ablation area. Control is provided by an iris diaphragm for the myopic portion of the correction and an adjustable slit aperture for the cylindrical portion of the correction. Both adjustable apertures are under computer control. A maximum of 240 individual positions allow a precise curve to be fit in where there is a predetermined number of the iris positions between each pulse. If only a few iris positions were available, then more pulses per positions would be required, and the "risers" of the steps would be taller.

Preoperative Management

Medication is given approximately 20 minutes prior to laser surgery. Preoperative medications include use of a nonsteroidal anti-inflammatory drop such as ketorolac tromethamine 0.5 % (Acular) or diclofenac sodium 0.1% (Voltaren), given one drop every 10 minutes for three times. These drops have shown to decrease postoperative pain. The use of an antibiotic

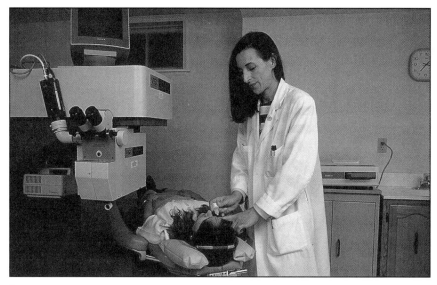

Figure 8-1. Topical anesthetic is administered preoperatively.

such as Ciloxan or Ocuflox are used to decrease the chance of any infection.

Immediately prior to laser surgery, several drops of a topical anesthetic (proparacaine hydrochloride) are instilled onto the eye (Figure 8-1). The patient is then positioned under the laser (Figure 8-2). A wire lid speculum is inserted. The non-operative eye is taped closed for comfort and better fixation of the eye to be ablated.

Eye Fixation

Centration is critical in achieving excellent visual results. The surgeon aligns the laser beam with the center of the entrance pupil, the virtual image of the pupil formed by the cornea, because centration of PRK relative to the center of the pupil decreases the chances of halos and/or glare, especially at night. There are four options to eye fixation:

1. **Fixation ring with suction**—A hand-held suction ring can be used to stabilize the globe. This device is usually large and cumbersome to use. It is relatively easy to put asymmetric pressure on the globe to distort the cornea. A new, disposable suction speculum, designed by Dr. Neal Sher, is easier to use and provides superior alignment.

2. **Fixation ring without suction**—There are a variety of fixation rings available. Types include the Barraquer, Gelender, and Katena rings. A small 10-mm Stein-Thornton compression ring redesigned by one of us (HAS) is easy to use and effective.

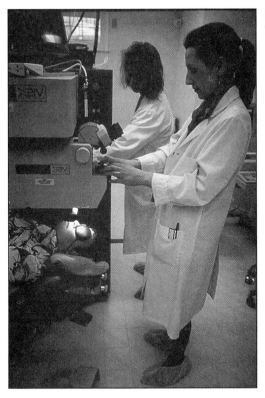

Figure 8-2. The patient is positioned beneath the laser.

3. **Forceps**—Not widely used because of an increased risk of discomfort, subconjunctival hemorrhage, and distortion of the globe.

4. **Self-fixation**—The majority of patients are able to cooperate and fixate on a target light. By turning down the operating microscope light and with indirect illumination, patient self-fixation is easier to achieve. Occasionally, external fixation is required, but self-fixation is currently our most popular method for the majority of patients.

With the VisX 20/20 B, in addition to concentrating through the dominant ocular of the microscope on the central portion of the pupil, we use a circle that is drawn on the screen for the centration. This will vary from time to time as we use a centering device to ablate a black film strip. We then identify this on the screen and draw a circle at that point. This usually will last for the day. While the surgeon is looking through the microscope, and in particular the dominant ocular of the microscope, the technician is watching the screen so that the eye is centered well in the circle (Figure 8-3). With the VisX STAR, the projected red reticule should be centered over the pupil.

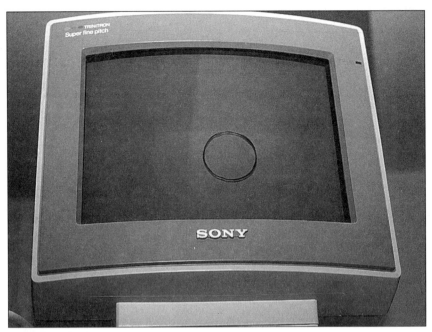

Figure 8-3. Centration circle drawn on the video monitor.

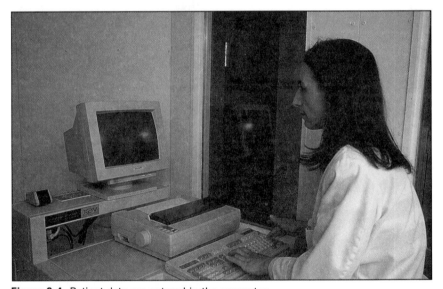

Figure 8-4. Patient data are entered in the computer.

Computer Inputting

Relevant data are entered into the computer (Figure 8-4). Depending on the laser and the available software, this may include name, date of birth, refraction, intended correction, keratometry values, epithelial removal

continued on page 75

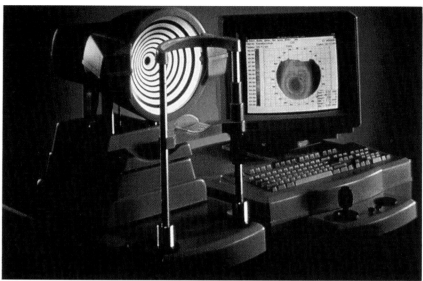

Figure 6-5. Videokeratoscopy unit showing illuminated keratoscopy rings and attached computer for digitization of both qualitative and quantitative data. Courtesy of EyeSys Co.

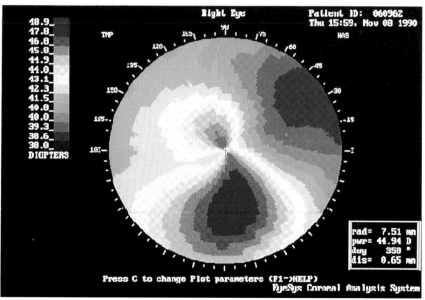

Figure 6-6. Videokeratoscope showing steepening inferiorly suggestive of keratoconus. This patient had clinical keratoconus with apical thinning and Vogt's striae.

See Chapter 6, <u>Videokeratography</u>, pages 52-58 for complete text accompanying these figures.

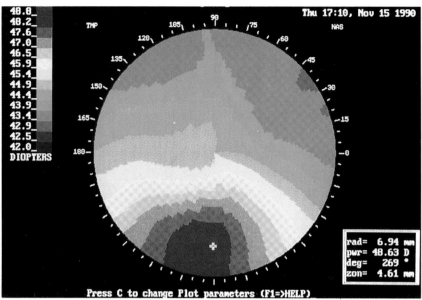

Figure 6-7. Videokeratoscope documenting a subtle form of keratoconus with inferior steepening. This patient had a normal slit lamp examination, keratometry mires, and refraction.

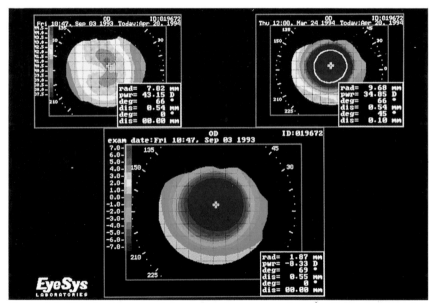

Figure 6-8. Videokeratoscope pictures showing preoperative map (left), postoperative map (right), and a difference map (below). Note the well-centered laser ablation.

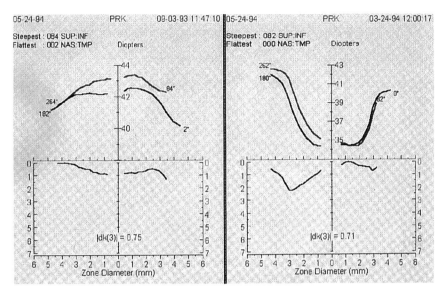

Figure 6-9. Profile drawing showing preoperative corneal contour (left) and post-PRK contour (right).

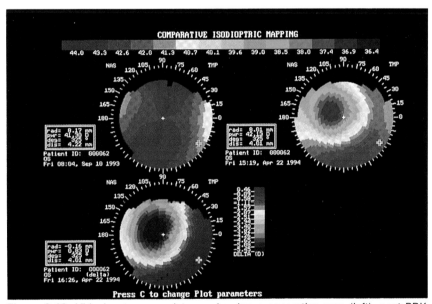

Figure 6-10. Videokeratoscope pictures showing preoperative map (left), post-PRK map (right), and a difference map (below). Note that the difference map shows evidence of decentration accounting for halos at nighttime.

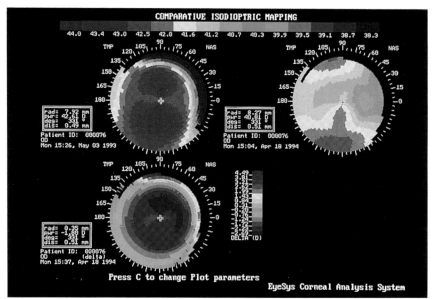

Figure 6-11. Videokeratoscope pictures showing preoperative map (left), post-PRK map (right), and a difference map (below). Note that the post-PRK pattern appears irregular; this is secondary to the preoperative asymmetric astigmatism.

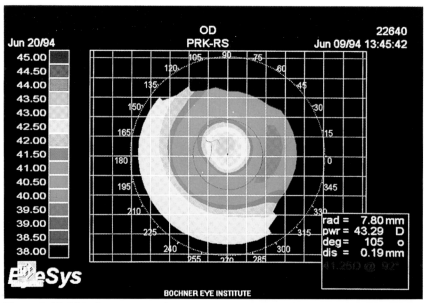

Figure 6-12. Videokeratoscope showing a central island 1 month postoperatively that was responsible for best-corrected acuity of 20/50. After 3 months, the island resolved and the patient had an uncorrected acuity of 20/20.

technique, optical zone, transition zone, single pass or multipass, single zone or multizone, and anti-island correction.

Epithelium Removal Technique

Different corneal tissues ablate at different rates, so the amount of tissue removed with each pulse varies. The cornea is not a homogeneous structure and the epithelium ablates at a faster rate than the corneal stroma. In a study in a donor eye model, the epithelium ablated at a rate of 0.68 ± 0.15 μm/pulse, and stroma ablated at a rate of 0.55 ± 0.1 μm/pulse.

Precise, quick epithelial removal is crucial to a good PRK outcome. A variety of removal techniques exist, and all have advantages and disadvantages from the surgeon's and patient's standpoints.

The epithelium can be removed by four methods (Figures 8-5A and 8-5B):

1. Mechanical debridement—sharp or blunt. Mechanical epithelial removal should not take longer than 2 minutes to avoid corneal hydration changes that may affect the outcome. Mechanical debridement consists of marking a 6- or 7-mm circular groove on the host corneal epithelium over the pupil, not the visual axis. A blunt paton spatula is used to scrape the epithelium from the periphery in toward the center (Figures 8-6A and 8-6B). A Weckcel sponge is soaked in a preservative-free artificial tear solution and wiped across the cornea. A spatula is used to remove excess fluid. The resultant "glistening" cornea is ideal for PRK because it is uniformly moist, thereby lessening haze.

Beginning surgeons often try to remove the central epithelium first, then struggle with the peripheral epithelium, exposing the central cornea to dehydration. This can result in overcorrection along with haze if one starts from the periphery. The quicker the epithelium is removed, the less chance for stromal dehydration.

The epithelium may be softened by repeated drops preoperatively. In most virgin corneas the epithelium comes away quite easily. In those patients who have had previous surgeries, such as RK, the epithelium is often found wedged between the grooves and is more difficult to remove. In any event, mechanical debridement is used by many as a satisfactory means of removing epithelium down to Bowman's layer, which provides a smooth anterior surface.

One advantage of this technique is that it is not dependent on the quality of the laser optics, as is the case in laser/scrape or transepithelial removal.

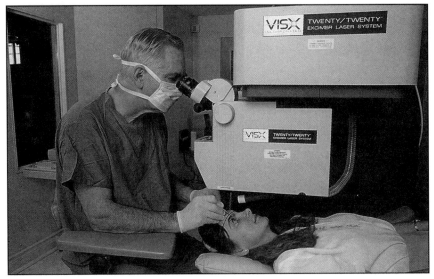

Figure 8-5A. The epithelium is removed.

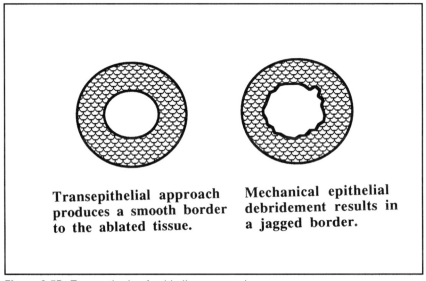

Transepithelial approach produces a smooth border to the ablated tissue.

Mechanical epithelial debridement results in a jagged border.

Figure 8-5B. Two methods of epithelium removal.

A disadvantage is that patients often prefer other techniques, such as transepithelial ablation. Also, the epithelium takes 1 to 2 days longer to heal. The surgeon should scrape from the outside in rather than inside out to avoid heaping the epithelium at the margins, which takes longer to heal.

2. Laser/scrape technique and transepithelial removal. Two laser removal approaches exist: the laser/scrape and the transepithelial technique.

The **laser/scrape** method is performed by typically removing 41 to 45

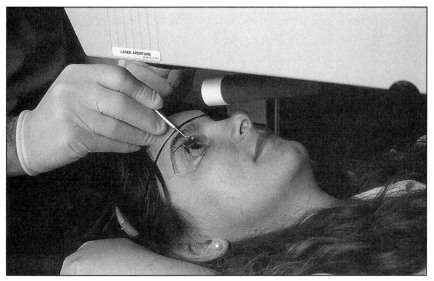

Figure 8-6A. Mechanical debridement of the epithelium.

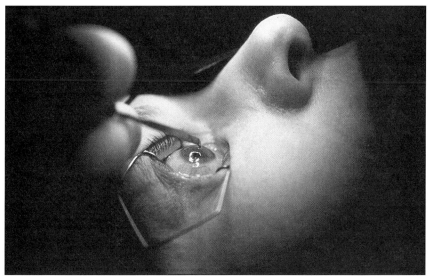

Figure 8-6B. Scrape the epithelium from the periphery in toward the center using a blunt paton spatula.

μm of tissue using a PTK ablation. The residual debris is mechanically removed with a spatula. This is relatively easy for beginning surgeons. Because the diaphragm is wide open, it is important to warn patients that the sound of the laser will be loud. If the PTK centration is not accurate, it makes stromal ablation hard to center.

This technique is dependent on the tear film quality, so once the lid speculum is inserted, the surgeon must proceed quickly. Waiting too long will cause tear film disruption and an irregular surface.

Patients with meibomitis and variable tear film quality may not be candidates for this technique.

Rather than using a standard depth for epithelial removal, another approach uses the blue fluorescence that appears when the laser strikes the epithelium. When the microscope light is dimmed, a blue fluorescence appears as the epithelium is ablated. Once the laser reaches the stroma, the blue fluorescence disappears, and the surgeon sees a black area. Typically, the peripheral stroma is reached before the center.

When the blue fluorescence disappears, the surgeon stops and scrapes the debris. It is not easy to detect when the blue fluorescence disappears; we do not typically use this approach for routine cases but for enhancements, especially if haze is present.

Although these epithelial defects heal faster than mechanical removal with a spatula, complications can occur with this method. If the stroma is entered too deeply, a steep border between unablated and ablated stroma results.

This can lead to an abnormal healing response with arcuate haze and scarring. Although this disappears with time, it can result in progressive hyperopia in that haze and scarring in the peripheral part of ablation will steepen the central cornea. Restarting the steroids is indicated in these hyperopic cases. In addition, arcuate haze may induce astigmatism. If this occurs, steroids should be restarted.

The pure **transepithelial laser** removal uses a 6-mm optical zone. Between 40 to 55 μm are used to ablate the epithelium; it varies in thickness. As the ablation is performed, a blue fluorescence is seen when the operating microscope light is turned down. When the epithelial ablation is complete and Bowman's layer is reached, the fluorescence disappears. There is a human variation of about 15 μm of epithelial thickness among individual corneas.

There has been some concern that there may not be uniformity across the width of the beam and that the laser may act more intensely in the periphery than the center.

Once the peripheral epithelium is removed, the surgeon notes the amount of microns necessary to go from that point through to the central epithelium. A nomogram can then be used to adjust the amount of correction required.

Although this no-touch technique is popular with patients, it increases the number of factors that affect outcomes; hence, it takes longer to master. It is

---

Table 8-1.
Technique for Alcohol Removal of the Epithelium

---

1. Open 10 cc ampule (Abbott) of absolute alcohol.
2. Dilute to 25% solution with BSS in sterile medicine cup (0.5 cc alcohol in 1.5 cc BSS).
3. Keep some solution in a 2-cc syringe for adding to additional cases. Solution may evaporate after 30 minutes and lose effect.
4. Soak a 6-mm absorbent Merocel disc (Mentor Occluder lens) in the medicine cup solution.
5. Place disc centrally on cornea for 3 minutes.
6. Rinse with cold BSS.
7. Lift epithelium with two McPherson forceps and tear apart. It will tear to outer ring ("epitheliorhexis") of the disc.
8. Rinse well again.
9. Begin ablation.

---

advantageous because the cornea is more uniformly moist.

3. Alcohol technique—the preferred method for one of us (HAS) is with diluted alcohol. Absolute alcohol is mixed with BSS to make a 25% solution and applied to a 6-mm Merocel disc. It is allowed to remain on the central cornea for 3 minutes. The central epithelium can then be lifted by two blunt McPherson forceps. Aron-Rosa claims the results are as good with this procedure as any other method of removing epithelium, and that it also defines the layers clearly (Table 8-1). We have performed a study in which we try to determine the visual outcome using the alcohol method as compared to other methods for epithelium removal. We were surprised that the average 6-month data show that alcohol was superior in most cases to other methods of epithelial removal. We were concerned that there may be some hydration effect or toxicity on Bowman's layer or on the stroma in cases of repeat PRK. None of these factors seem to be a problem. Our outcome analysis showed that 67% using alcohol achieved 20/20 vision and the majority achieved 20/25. There were no cases that were any worse than 20/40 within 6 months. Thus, alcohol is a good method for removal of the epithelium. It leaves Bowman's layer crystal clear for ablation. In cases of scraping, there is always some slight microscopic residual epithelium left on the cornea or small divots induced by the scraping. None is the case with 25% alcohol removal.

Another technique uses a 6- or 7-mm metal optical zone marker placed on the eye and a few drops of 20% alcohol placed within the marker. After 20 to

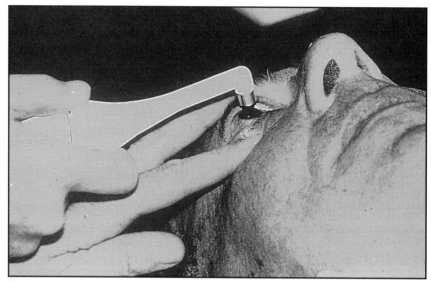

Figure 8-7. Rotary brush technique of Drs. Amoils and Pallikaris.

30 seconds, the alcohol is irrigated and the epithelium comes off easily.

By using this approach, the epithelium usually heals within 2 to 3 days with minimal transient corneal haze.

4. The rotary brush (Figure 8-7) as developed by Drs. Percy Amoils and Ioannis Pallikaris consists of a rotary brush which removes the epithelium. It has fine hairs that do not injure the underlying Bowman's layer. This provides a smooth corneal surface.

The rotary brush, modified by Amoils and distributed by Innova (Toronto, Canada), is a relatively new modality that has recently received US FDA approval. To effectively remove epithelium, the brush has been modified with a specially designed collar to shorten bristle length. There are 6- and 9-mm brushes.

This technique is easy; the epithelium is removed in a few seconds. This appears to be promising, especially for hyperopic ablations, which generally require removing 9 mm of epithelium, a procedure that is too lengthy and difficult with spatula removal. It is important to use a rotary, not an oscillating, brush to achieve complete epithelial removal.

A disadvantage is that patients lose fixation when the pupil is occluded with the brush, and, due to eye movement, the surgeon can remove too much epithelium. Disposable sterile brushes are available that make this a very attractive technique.

Other Issues

Because it excessively dried the cornea, nitrogen blowing is no longer used. Often it caused differential drying; its use resulted in a high incidence of haze and, therefore, was abandoned. Although haze occurred, there were no cases of central islands.

The VisX 20/20 B and STAR models use a suction tube placed about 1.25 inches away from cornea, and all nomograms are based on this device. Therefore, this distance must be verified. If the suction tube is too close to the eye, it will dehydrate the corneal surface, resulting in overcorrections. If it is too far away, fluid will accumulate, resulting in undercorrections.

Summit Technology's SVS Apex Plus excimer laser does not use suction tubes; therefore, the internal nomograms reflect this state.

Theoretically, room humidity may affect outcomes. As surgeons develop their own data pool, it is important to keep as many factors as possible constant. That means keeping temperature and humidity relatively constant in the laser room. It is worthwhile keeping temperature and humidity gauges there. In our experience, a cornea that is too dry after epithelial removal and/or during laser ablation may result in haze.

Stromal Ablation

A precise amount of tissue can be removed with each pulse of the laser, which depends on the energy level of the laser beam. An average 0.25 µm of tissue can be ablated per pulse of the laser so that four pulses ablate 1 µm. Each photon has an extremely high energy level of approximately 6.4 eV. This level is higher than that holding the corneal molecules together, which is 3.4 eV. When the laser beam makes contact with the cornea, the intermolecular bonds are broken and the molecules are dispersed into the air at a rate of 2000 m/sec. This process leaves a clear and smooth underlying corneal surface (Figure 8-8).

An important concern is corneal stroma hydration. The depth ablated per pulse could be increased if the cornea is less hydrated, so the eye would be overcorrected. If the cornea is too hydrated, an undercorrection can occur.

Cold Balance Saline

We have found that cold balance saline placed on the cornea following the procedure or after each of the multipass or multizone ablations cools the cornea and provides clearer corneas. If irrigating after each multipass or multizone ablation we allow the cornea to dry slightly just before beginning the next stage of the ablation process, it is not dehydrated. We feel that dehydration contributes significantly to haze. We also feel that cooling the cornea slightly with cold balance salt taken from the refrigerator reduces

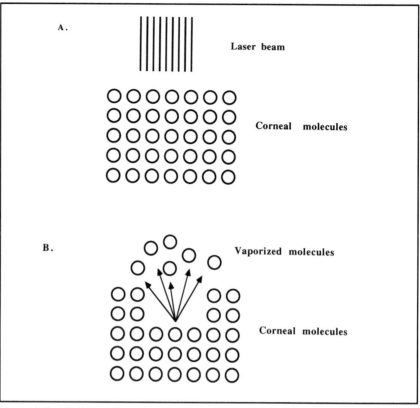

Figure 8-8. (A) PRK with the excimer laser is possible because of the high energy of the laser beam. (B) The laser results in the breakage of intermolecular bonds and the vaporization of molecules leaving the underlying surface relatively unaffected.

any microscopic debris that may have fallen onto the cornea during the ablation process and makes the patient more comfortable when wearing a bandage lens.

In order to induce a myopic refractive change, more tissue has to be removed from the center of the cornea than the periphery (Figure 8-9), which is achieved by a diaphragm system that opens initially from the center and then out to the periphery (Figure 8-10). By this technique, more laser light hits the center of the cornea than the peripheral aspects of the ablation, resulting in a refractive change.

The larger the optical zone, the more tissue that has to be removed for a given refractive error. For example, if one were to choose a 3-mm optical zone to correct -10 D, the central depth of ablation would be 30 μm. If a 6-mm optical zone were chosen, the central depth of ablation would be approximately 120 μm (Figure 8-11).

The problem with small optical zones is that if the pupil dilates,

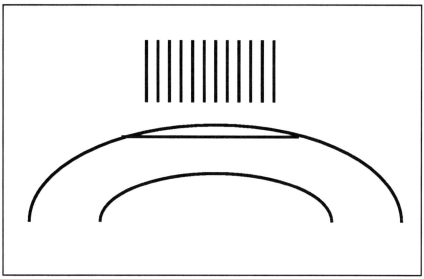

Figure 8-9. More tissue is removed from the central cornea than the peripheral part of the ablation. This results in the correction of a myopic refractive error.

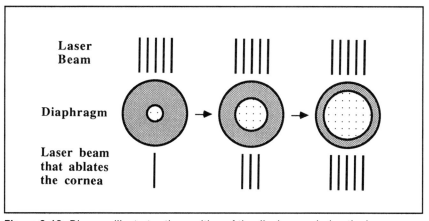

Figure 8-10. Diagram illustrates the position of the diaphragm during the laser procedure. Note that the central cornea receives more laser than the peripheral cornea.

especially at night, halos can be produced as a result of refraction of light at the edge of the ablation. In addition, small optical zones are associated with regression as the epithelium attempts to fill in the divot created by the laser.

The larger the optical zone, the easier it is for the surgeon to center the treatment over the pupil. One can imagine playing a game of darts and having a dart the size of the dart board. The chances of hitting the bull's eye would be excellent.

The central depth of ablation (μm) is equal to the refractive change (D) divided by three and then multiplied by the optical zone (mm) squared.

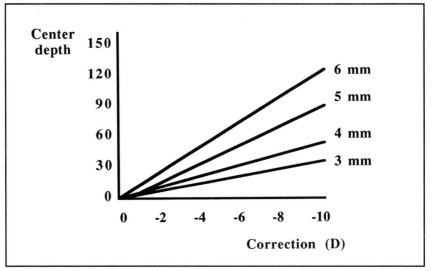

Figure 8-11. Effective depth (μm) of corneal ablation at different optical zone diameters (mm).

	Table 8-2. Intended Correction (D) vs. Central Depth of Ablation (μm)	
	Central Depth of Ablation	
Intended Correction	*5 mm*	*6 mm*
-1.00 D	8.3 μm	12.0 μm
-2.00 D	16.6	24.0
-3.00 D	25.0	36.0
-4.00 D	33.3	48.0
-5.00 D	41.6	60.0
-6.00 D	50.0	72.0

$$\text{central depth of ablation (μm)} = \frac{\text{refractive change (D)}}{3} \times \text{optical zone}^2 \text{(mm)}$$

This formula allows calculation of the central depth of the ablation given the intended refractive change and the optical zone selected (Table 8-2). The amount of tissue removed is generally minimal. For example, for -2 D at 6 mm, 24 μm of tissue are removed. With a -6 D intended correction with a 6-mm optical zone, 72 μm of tissue are ablated.

The correction of astigmatism is achieved by a diaphragm system that opens with a slit and then opens all the way to a sphere. As the iris slit gradually opens, a flattening occurs in the direction of the opening of the slit. There is no refractive change that occurs in the opposite meridian (see

Figures 13-3A and 13-3B).

There are three components to the stromal ablation:

1. Pretreatment to prevent central islands
2. Astigmatism correction
3. Spherical correction

Pretreatment

Currently, pretreatment is performed to prevent the development of central islands. When central islands occur they are represented postoperatively by an elevated spot in the center of the cornea that is usually <2 1/2 mm in size. On computerized topography, it is referred to as a hot spot since the warmer colors represent an area of steepness. The etiology of these central islands is not well understood, but a number of possibilities exist:

- Shockwaves push fluid to the center of the cornea during the procedure, and this fluid blocks the laser beam in the center so it does not get as much ablation
- The plume or vaporized molecules over the cornea may block the laser beam
- Optical degradation
- Epithelial hyperplasia (thickening) occurs postoperatively

To prevent central islands, we currently use a pretreatment of 1 µm/D of correction using a 2.5-mm optical zone. For example, if one were to treat -6 D, one would use 6 µm at 2 1/2 mm. By removing these additional microns at the center of the cornea, the finding of central islands is rare. If central islands occur they usually disappear over a period of 4 to 8 months.

Astigmatism

With the VisX 20/20 B or STAR excimer lasers, astigmatism can be treated either in an elliptical module or a sequential module. It is preferable to use the elliptical module as results are superior, but one is restricted to cases in which the sphere is greater than or equal to the astigmatism (eg, -3.00 -2.00 x 180). If the sphere is less than the astigmatism (eg, -0.50 -2.00 x 180), then a sequential mode is used in which the astigmatism is treated first and then the sphere. With the elliptical module, both the astigmatism and the sphere are treated at the same time.

Spherical Correction

There are a variety of approaches to the treatment of myopia. Depending on the available software, one can perform a single zone with a single pass, a single zone with multipasses, a multizone with single passes, or a multizone and multipass.

Munnerlyn's law states that the central depth of the ablation in microns is equal to the refractive change in diopters divided by three times the square of the optical zone in millimeters. Hence, the depth of the ablation in microns rises exponentially with the diameter of the optic zone squared. The whole purpose with a multizone approach is to reduce the depth of the ablation. There are marked differences in visual outcome when using a multizone technique. Corneas are clearer with shallower ablations.

The degree of intended correction determines the optical zone size that is chosen. For refractive errors of ≤6 D, a single 6-mm optical zone is chosen. Between 6 D and 10 D, two optical zones are chosen in which 60% of the correction is performed at 5 mm and 40% at 6 mm. For corrections of >10 D, three optical zones are chosen in which 50% of the correction is performed at 4.5 mm, 30% at 5 mm, and 20% at 6 mm (Figures 8-12A and 8-12B). There are a significant number of variations that can be chosen (ie, number and size of optical zones).

By performing multiple zones of correction, the depth of ablation is decreased. For example, if one were to treat -15 D using a single 6-mm optical zone, one would ablate 196 μm. If one were to use a three-zone technique, then 122 μm of tissue would be ablated. Multiple zones also produce a smoother transition between the edge of the ablation and surrounding tissue, leading to decreased corneal haze and regression.

With a multizone technique, there is an analog to contact lens technology in that one is producing a peripheral blend and hence the depth of the ablation is greatly diminished.

With multipass technique, we get smoother zones by virtue of normal saccadic movement and slight decentration of the laser beam with each pass that is unintentional. This results in less haze and regression. For example, in doing a single pass in a 6 D myope, one can see rings or terraces which coincide with the openings of the iris diaphragm. After a few passes, the rings tend to disappear and the surface appears smoother.

Generally, each pass of the laser can be programmed to treat a low degree of myopia. One approach is to establish a specific number of zones and then treat each zone with passes of no more than 2 D.

Short intervals between each pass allow the cornea to cool sufficiently, which may be responsible for less corneal haze. It is possible to irrigate between passes with cold BSS and wipe slightly dry with a cellulose sponge. This may have the effect of further decreasing corneal temperature and hydrating a dry cornea.

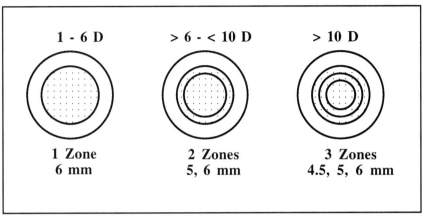

Figure 8-12A. Diagrams depicting the zones of treatment for low, moderate, and high myopia.

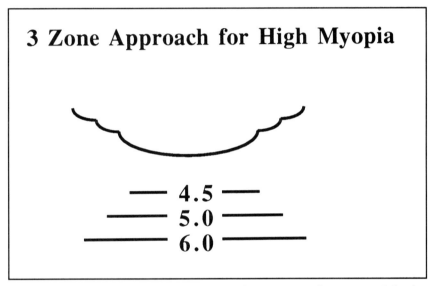

Figure 8-12B. Cross-section of the cornea showing exaggerated appearance following a three-zone approach in the treatment of high myopia

In conclusion, a combination of multizone and multipass gives the best visual results with a broad beam excimer laser and results in a much quicker attainment of ultimate visual acuity with less regression and less haze than occurred when using a single ablation technique.

Centration Key to Good PRK Outcomes

Decentered ablations are best approached from a preventative standpoint because, to date, no satisfactory treatment exists. It is important to center the ablation over the pupil and not the visual axis when using a 6-mm optical zone. If a patient has a positive or negative angle kappa and the surgeon centers on the visual axis, the ablation will be decentered relative to the pupil, a situation that could result in glare and halos, especially at night.

Additionally, the surgeon should focus on the surface of the cornea. This is important when using certain lasers; the Summit Apex, for example, must be focused. Most of the other lasers have colluminated beams that do not require focusing.

Focusing on the corneal surface helps with centration. If the surgeon is focused at the iris level, it can be difficult to determine if the eye is tilted. One can be focused in the center of the pupil, at the level of the iris, and actually be ablating the superior portion of the cornea.

Holding, Fixation

Several years ago, researchers at VisX believed that holding the globe with an instrument would provide better centration than relying on the patient to self-fixate. In our hands, however, self-fixation results in better centration.

When the surgeon holds the eye, it is easy to put undue pressure on one quadrant or another, thereby distorting the globe. The patient is best suited to stare at the red fixation light.

Occasionally, patients are unable to concentrate or are unable to see the fixation light. In these cases, we resort to holding the globe. Treating higher corrections is more difficult because patients have more trouble fixating as the corneal surface dries during the procedure.

The VisX STAR laser and others that use an indirect illumination system make it much easier for patients to look at the fixation light. The pupil is well illuminated by the light shining through the normal clear cornea, not through the ablated cornea.

Eye Trackers

Several laser companies (Chiron Vision, Autonomous Technologies, Novatec Laser Systems, Nidek, and LaserSight Technologies) are developing eye tracking systems. These systems must track in x, y, and z planes; if the laser tracks only in the x-y plane and the patient's chin tilts up or down, alignment will be disrupted because the eye will be elevated or depressed.

Preoperative Sedation

Preoperative sedation is indicated only if the surgeon plans on holding the eye during ablation. Preoperative sedation, therefore, is not recommended to avoid self-fixation problems.

Communicate

It is important to encourage your patients during the procedure, as patient/physician communication alleviates much patient anxiety. Patients may become concerned because their sight blurs during the procedure. It is important for the surgeon or assistant to talk to patients during the procedure to let them know they are doing well and to inform them that their vision will blur.

Some patients have panicked when their vision blurred because they thought they were losing their sight. Now we talk the patient through the entire process. Encouraging patients to relax helps ensure a good outcome.

Quiet Please

For the patient to concentrate well, distractions should be kept to a minimum (ie, nursing staff and visiting doctors should not talk during the procedure). Patients listen in on the conversation and consequently their eyes may move.

Training

Training patients prior to laser surgery may be helpful. Some surgeons perform several pulses through the epithelium with the PTK protocol, which helps patients to become familiar with the sound of the laser. At the Beacon Eye Institute, a training flashlight has been designed that simulates the laser light. Training with this instrument may improve patient concentration and therefore the final visual outcome.

Topography

Corneal videokeratoscopy should be performed preoperatively and at 1 month postoperative, and the difference maps should be evaluated. Preoperative topographies, therefore, are essential to derive the difference map postoperatively. At 1 month, the difference will tell whether the ablation has been properly centered. This feedback allows the surgeon to monitor and improve centration techniques, especially in patients who are asymptomatic, with small pupils, and a mildly decentered ablation.

Summary

Following a strict routine prior to surgery is absolutely necessary. Table 8-3 outlines the steps that should be performed with each surgery.

Some material adapted from Stein R. Quick epithelial removal key to good outcomes. *OSN*. 1996;May 15:33.

Table 8-3.
PRK Procedure for Myopia and Astigmatism

Safety Checks
Correct patient, correct eye determined
Fluence level determined
Ablate plastic
Ablate a piece of plastic or paper to check centration

Preoperative Management
Medication 20 minutes before surgery; one drop every 10 minutes times 3
- Nonsteroidal drop (eg, Acular or Voltaren)
- Antibiotic (eg, Ciloxan, Ocuflox, etc)
- Steroid (eg, FML, Flarex, etc)

Patient is placed upright in the chair and the chair leveled
Nonoperative eye is covered
Headrest is placed in position to minimize movement
Several drops of a topical anesthetic are instilled (eg, proparacine)

Surgical Procedure
Lid speculum is inserted
Center of patient's pupil is aligned under microscope
Epithelium is removed
Pretreatment to prevent central islands
Astigmatism correction with elliptical or sequential program
Spherical correction
Lid speculum removed

Immediate Postoperative Management
Drops instilled: nonsteroidal, antibiotic, and/or steroid
Insertion of disposable bandage soft contact lens
Postoperative medication and instructions given
Patient to be seen the next day

Chapter 9

Postoperative Management

With PRK, transitory changes in visual acuity are frequently observed postoperatively. These visual changes correspond with changes in corneal transparency and corneal topography. It is essential that the patient understand these temporary changes may occur.

Immediately postoperatively, a drop of a nonsteroidal anti-inflammatory (eg, Acular or Voltaren), a drop of topical antibiotic, and a drop of a topical steroid are instilled. The combination of pre- and postoperative nonsteroidal along with a contact lens has resulted in such a major decrease in pain that now 90% of the patients have essentially no discomfort following laser surgery. The 10% who do have discomfort have usually minimal discomfort overnight which quickly resolves. Prior to the use of nonsteroidal drops, all patients had significant pain. This important breakthrough in treatment is thought to be related to the blockage of prostaglandins by the nonsteroidals and the protective effect of the contact lens on the denuded epithelial surface.

The disposable bandage contact lens should be inserted at the time of laser surgery (Figure 9-1) and removed when the epithelial defect is healed, which usually occurs in 2 to 3 days.

First Week Postoperatively

In the first 3 days, follow-up examinations are scheduled at 24-hour intervals or until the epithelium is healed. Anti-inflammatory drops (Acular or Voltaren) are instilled five times a day while awake for 2 days. An antibiotic (eg, Ciloxan, Ocuflox) is used five times a day for 5 days. A corticosteroid is instilled five times a day while awake and slowly tapered.

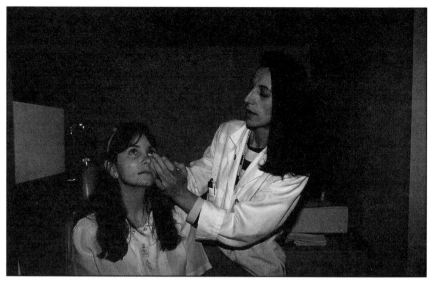

Figure 9-1. A disposable bandage contact lens is inserted.

This will be discussed below.

Re-epithelialization usually takes 2 to 3 days. On the second or third day the bandage contact lens is usually removed. If the contact lens is removed prior to epithelial healing, the patient will often experience significant pain.

Steroid Course

There is no universally accepted steroid regimen. Reasonable options consist of one of the follow:

1. **No steroid**—If during follow-up there is significant regression or haze, then steroids are started.

2. **Short steroid course**—For example, the steroids can be used four times a day for 1 week, three times a day for 1 week, two times a day for 1 week, then once a day for 1 week. If there is overcorrection, regression, or significant haze, then the steroid dosage and course can be altered.

3. **Long steroid course**—The topical steroid can be used five times a day for 1 month, four times a day for 1 month, three times a day for 1 month, twice a day for 1 month, then finally once a day for 1 month. This regimen may be altered if overcorrection, regression, or significant haze develops (Table 9-1).

Table 9-1.
Patient Discharge Instructions

Activity
The first 12 to 24 hours may be uncomfortable. The amount of discomfort each patient experiences is variable. You may be sensitive to bright light. The more you use your treated eye, the more discomfort you may experience. Watching TV or reading may be done in moderation. Do not drive a car while you are taking pain medication.

Dressings
Keep the treated eye protected while outside (wear sunglasses). Showers are permitted but do not get the eye wet. If the bandage contact lens falls out during the night, do not insert the lens, but continue administering the eyedrops. The surface (epithelial) cells heal during the first 48 to 72 hours, during which time your vision may be very blurry and the eye will feel itchy. The eye may tear and be red and swollen. These are normal postoperative symptoms and will disappear within a few days. The contact lens is to remain in your eye until your return appointment with the doctor.

Eyedrops
Nonsteroidal (Acular or Voltaren): One drop every 3 hours while awake, taken for 2 days
Antibiotic (Ciloxan or Ocuflox): One drop every 3 hours while awake, taken for 5 days
Steroid (FML, FML forte, or Vexol): One drop every 3 hours while awake, taken for 1 month and then tapered
These drops will be used for approximately 1 to 6 months (the number of drops may be altered depending on your rate of healing).

Medications
Tylenol #3: One tablet every 3 to 4 hours for pain, only if needed (possible side effects are drowsiness and/or nausea)
Valium: a mild tranquilizer—one tablet if needed
Flurazepam: a sleeping pill—one tablet if needed
Separate the drops by 3 minutes.
Your vision will improve slowly and you may return to your normal activities of daily living after 3 to 4 days. Depth perception may be affected in the beginning as your eye heals. That is, you will find that your focus will vary throughout the day and it will take several seconds for objects to become clear. Your near vision will be especially blurry until the eye heals. It is important to remember that everyone has his or her own rate of healing—please be patient.

Drugs provided to patient.

Effect of Postoperative Steroids

The use of topical steroids post-PRK is controversial. Studies in the low myopia range (<6 D) have shown no significant difference in refractive outcome or development of haze between eyes treated with steroids and those treated with artificial tears. Our own clinical experience, especially in the high myope, is that there is greater evidence of regression and haze when steroids are not used or when they are discontinued abruptly. The answer to this controversy is not resolved at the time of this writing. We are hopeful that better and more effective nonsteroidal modulating medication will be developed by the pharmaceutical industry.

The use of topical corticosteroids following excimer laser surgery is widespread. This use is controversial because the role of corticosteroids remains poorly defined.

Because corticosteroids inhibit the stromal production of hyaluronic acid by keratocytes that are responsible for regression of the induced refractive change months after PRK, it has been argued that their use may reduce regression and haze formation. Disadvantages of this use are adverse effects, such as elevated IOP, posterior subcapsular cataracts, ptosis, and reactivation of herpes simplex keratitis.

The response of wound healing following excimer laser treatment is different for each patient. Wound healing can be generally classified into the following groups:
- Group I: normal healers
- Group II: inadequate healers
- Group III: strong healers

Patients from Group I have a normal refractive outcome. Group II patients never acquire the expected healing and are hyperopic. For this reason, the steroids are rapidly tapered in these patients. In Group III, there is a great amount of regression, so steroids are increased. These patients will frequently require secondary procedures.

The analysis of healing for each patient can be determined during the first few months after surgery by examining under slit lamp for corneal haze, refraction, and computerized videokeratography.

Effect of Nonsteroidal Anti-Inflammatories

Nonsteroidal anti-inflammatories, such as diclofenac sodium (Voltaren) and ketorolac tromethamine (Acular), through inhibition of prostaglandin synthesis, produce a potent analgesic effect that is very important in the early postoperative period following photorefractive surgery.

The use of diclofenac sodium has been shown to promote regression and therefore is occasionally used when dealing with an overcorrected PRK.

Dr. Neal Sher feels that the use of nonsteroidals should be combined with a topical steroid to prevent accumulation of white blood cells into the cornea, which produce corneal infiltrates. These infiltrates have been reported by Pat Teal in approximately 1 of 250 eyes in which steroids are not used with a nonsteroidal in the early postoperative period. A combination of steroids used with a nonsteroidal in the early postoperative period has prevented any corneal infiltrates in our last 3000 eyes since we have been using steroids and nonsteroids immediately following surgery.

Summary

The technical aspect is a precise technique beginning with a well-functioning excimer laser, good optics, and proper computer input. Safety checks are mandatory. The surgeon must avoid any decentration or global tilt. All aspects of the technique must be performed with attention to detail. The postoperative management requires frequent follow-up visits and psychological reinforcement of a healing process that is not instantaneous.

Results

Chapter 10

Photorefractive Keratectomy Results

Excimer laser use has had an exponential growth on an international level. It is estimated that at the time of this writing there have been over 1 million cases of PRK performed worldwide. In Canada during the past 6 years, there have been 55 units installed and operating in major cities, with an average of five physicians at each center. Backed in large part by business interests, excimers are correcting an estimated 1000 myopes each month in Canada. Data have been accumulating that document the safety, predictability, and stability of PRK.

The growing use of the excimer laser for PRK in Canada has led to a great deal of learning and shared experience that have enhanced the safety and comfort of the procedure. Canadian surgeons, not confined to a fixed protocol for PRK, have been able to make modifications in excimer use that have lessened several associated complications, making PRK safer and the outcome better. For example:

- Blowing nitrogen to keep the cornea dry was found to cause complications with increased haze and was promptly abandoned.
- The use of ketorolac tromethamine (Acular) and diclofenac sodium (Voltaren) has significantly reduced postoperative pain. Following surgery, a bandage soft contact lens is placed on the eye and patients are given the drops to minimize postoperative discomfort.
- Patient management has been better understood.
- Patient selection has been better defined.
- Risks have been more appreciated.
- Prevention and management of central islands have improved.
- The variable delay in full recovery of uncorrected vision has become better understood.

- The timing and technique of retreatment have been better understood.
- More complications have been seen and better managed.

Dr. Richard Lindstrom said, "Clearly the excimer laser appears to have efficacy in the -1.00 D to -6.00 D group. If we treat higher degrees of myopia, that efficacy falls off. But in the most recent studies we have been achieving 80% to 90% of patients seeing 20/40 or better, and as many as 70% or 80% of them seeing 20/30 or better with one treatment. The efficacy of the laser appears to have become established" (personal communication, 1996).

The results of recent studies (Gartry et al, Salz et al, Tengroth et al) on myopia from 1 D to 6 D have been excellent, with more than 90% of eyes achieving uncorrected visual acuities better than 20/40.

Kim et al evaluated the results of PRK on 45 consecutive eyes with a range from -2.00 D to -6.00 D. Uncorrected visual acuity better than 20/25 was achieved in 88.9% of all cases 2 years postoperatively. The difference between the attempted and achieved correction was within ±1.00 D in 91.1% 2 years postoperatively.

Talley et al evaluated the results of PRK on 91 sighted patients with preoperative refractive errors that have ranged from -1.00 D to -7.50 D with a mean of -4.11 D. At 6 months, 93% of eyes were within 1.00 D of attempted correction, 93% had uncorrected visual acuity of 20/40 or better, and 72% achieved uncorrected visual acuity of 20/25 or better. All patients returned to within one line of their preoperative best-corrected visual acuity.

In the early clinical studies of PRK by Gartry et al and Seiler et al, it was theorized that deep ablations would result in significant corneal haze or scarring. Therefore, the clinical approach to treating higher levels of myopia was to use smaller ablation zones. In these early studies, investigators found significant regression and corneal haze. McDonald et al postulated that the smaller ablation diameters led to relatively steep edges resulting in a healing response in the stroma that filled in the ablation.

Sher et al reported results with a 5-mm optical zone and intensive topical steroids on seven sighted eyes with myopia ranging from -5.5 D to -12.0 D. This study showed that PRK was capable of reducing larger amounts of myopia without serious haze or regression. Since this study there have been numerous reports (Brancato et al, Buratto & Ferrari, Cho et al, Ehlers & Hjortdal, Kim et al, Lavery, Sher et al) showing success of the excimer laser in treating high levels of myopia with a larger single optical zone, although there has been considerable variation in the results with undercorrection, overcorrection, and regression still of concern.

Trokel and colleagues suggested a two-zone approach using 5- and 6-mm optical zones. In 1992, a protocol for two-zone (60% of correction at 5 mm, 40% at 6 mm) and three-zone ablations (50% of correction at 4 mm, 30% at 5 mm, and 20% at 6 mm) was started using the VisX 20/20 B machine. The advantage of a multizone technique is that the depth of ablation can be reduced by 30% to 40%.

In 1993, Heitzmann and coworkers published the results of a multizone (4.0, 5.0, and 6.0 mm) PRK protocol for correction of high myopia, 23 eyes in 18 patients. Preoperative spherical equivalent refractions ranged from -8.00 D to -19.50 D (mean ±SD, -11.83 D ±2.92 D). At the last postoperative examination (mean ±SD, -7.5 D ±3.7 months), the mean ±SD spherical equivalent refraction was -1.09 D ±2.08 D, including results from two repeated procedures. Visual acuity was 20/40 or better uncorrected in 52% of the eyes; 65% of the eyes improved or did not change best-corrected acuity, whereas two eyes lost two Snellen lines; 39% of the eyes were ±1.00 D; and 65% were ± 2.00 D of attempted correction. Corneal haze (corneal clarity score of ≥1.5 D) was observed in 47% of the eyes at some time postoperatively.

PRK for myopic astigmatism has been demonstrated to be an effective means for the treatment of astigmatism (Dausch et al, McDonnell et al, Pender, Spigelman et al). A cylindrical ablation can be achieved by using either a slit-shaped or an elliptical beam. Data on the treatment of astigmatism are often difficult to interpret as it is often discussed in terms of a spheroequivalent and not on the amount of astigmatism corrected. Spigelman et al showed in 70 patients that cylinder was reduced from an average of -1.52 D to -0.54 D 6 months postoperatively. At 1 year, the average preoperative cylinder was reduced from -1.19 D to -0.59 D in 12 patients. Adjustments in nomograms are being made to improve the accuracy and predictability. Chapter 11 discusses the treatment of astigmatism in more detail.

Bochner Eye Institute Results

At the time of this writing we have performed excimer laser on more than 6000 eyes with long follow-ups since 1991. We have reviewed our first 3000 treated eyes at the Bochner Eye Institute (Table 10-1). All of these procedures were performed by us. Of the first 1000 eyes, 840 eyes were treated with PRK and 160 eyes with PTK (Figure 10-1).

Of the PRK group there were 609 eyes with mild myopia (<6.00 D), 137

Table 10-1.
PRK Results: 3000 Eyes

20/40 or Better Uncorrected Visual Acuity

	First 1000 Eyes	*Second 1000 Eyes*	*Third 1000 Eyes*
1 D to <6 D	95%	96%	97%
6 D to <10 D	77%	78%	83%
10 D to 15 D	65%	72%	78%

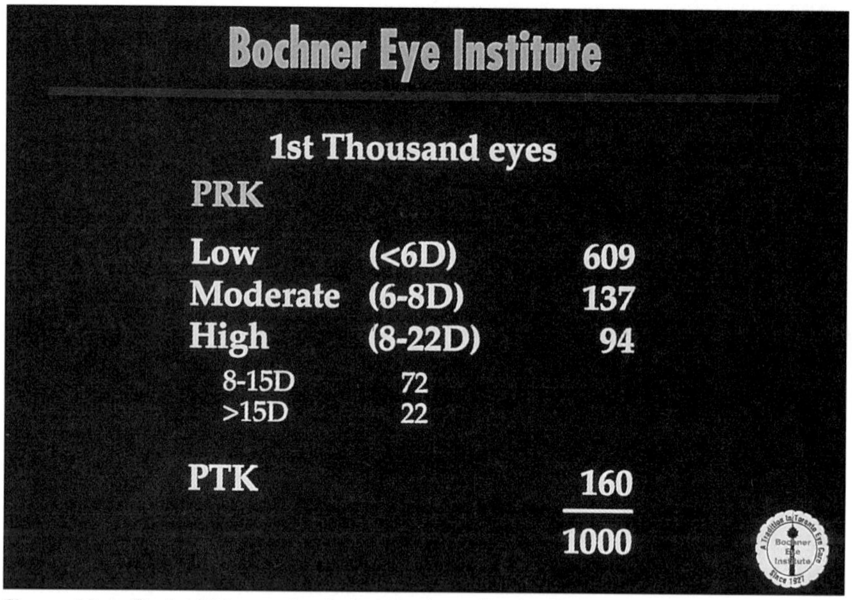

Figure 10-1. First 1000 eyes treated at Bochner Eye Institute.

eyes with moderate myopia (between 6.00 D and 8.00 D), and 94 eyes with myopia >8.00 D. Of the 94 eyes >8.00 D, there were 72 eyes between 8.00 D and 15.00 D and 22 eyes >15.00 D (Figure 10-2).

The technique of epithelial removal changed during the course of the study. In the first 1000 eyes, approximately 50% had mechanical epithelial removal and 50% had laser plus scrape. There did not appear to be a statistically significant difference in outcome with these two different epithelial removal techniques. In recognized cases of anterior basement membrane dystrophy, a mechanical debridement of the epithelium was performed to decrease the possibility of inducing irregular astigmatism.

To prevent central islands, the technique of pretreatment was used over the past 6 years. In this technique (see Chapter 8), after the epithelium has been removed, 1 µm/D of intended correction is ablated using a 2.5-mm

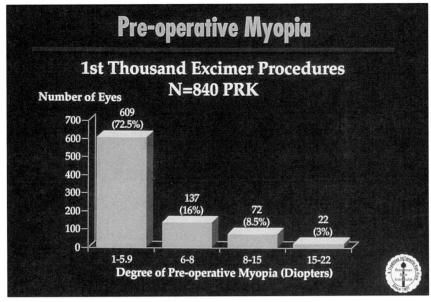

Figure 10-2. PRK results.

optical zone. After this pretreatment was done, the spherical and astigmatic ablation was performed.

For myopia between 6 D and <10 D, the spherical stromal ablations were done with two ablation zones with each programmed such that 60% of the correction was performed at 5 mm and 40% at 6 mm. This dual zone effectively decreases the depth of ablation. For myopia of ≥10 D, multi-zones were performed. Three optical zones were chosen initially such that 50% of the ablation was performed at 4.5 mm, 30% at 5 mm, and 20% at 6 mm (Figure 10-3). Accurate centration, especially in these patients, is more difficult because the patient has more difficulty seeing the target and because of the longer time required for fixation during the three steps. External fixation, although generally uncommon, was occasionally required to stabilize the eye.

Our initial results show that with myopia between 1.00 D and <6.00 D, 95% of the patients achieve 20/40 or better acuity; between 6.00 D and 8.00 D, 85% of patients achieve 20/40 or better acuity; and >8.00 D to 22.00 D, 72.6% of the patients achieve 20/40 or better acuity. Of the patients that were undercorrected, additional laser therapy achieved good visual results. Overall, with one or more laser procedures, 90% of patients obtain a visual acuity of 20/25 or better, and 98% achieve 20/40 or better.

Eighty percent of the mild myopia cases were within 0.5 D of emmetropia and 95% were within 1.0 D (Figure 10-4). Of the moderate

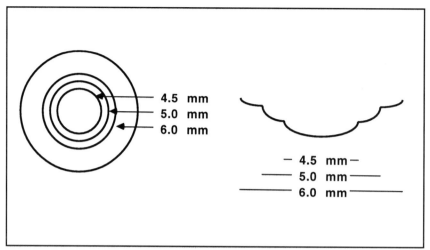

Figure 10-3. Three optical zones.

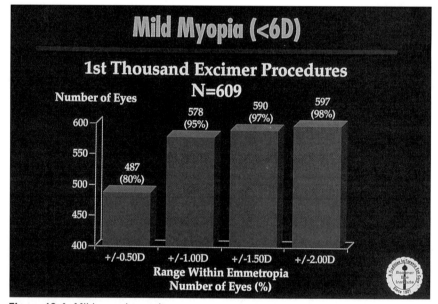

Figure 10-4. Mild myopia results.

myopia cases, 74% were within 0.5 D of emmetropia, while 85% were within 1.0 D (Figure 10-5). In the high myopia group, only 47% of cases were within 0.5 D of emmetropia while 72.6% were within 1.0 D (Figure 10-6).

Figures 10-7 through 10-9 show the mean refraction over time for the three groups. All three groups achieved an improved correction, with some regression over time. The high myopia group experienced the most regression with stability generally occurring between 6 and 12 months.

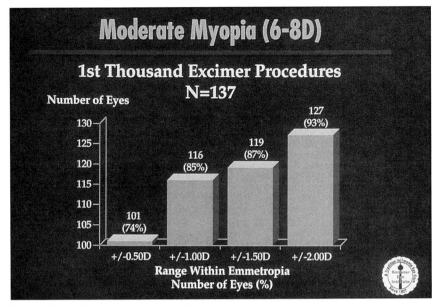

Figure 10-5. Moderate myopia results.

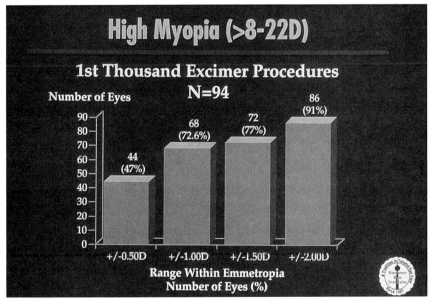

Figure 10-6. High myopia results.

The correction of astigmatism was approached with the sequential module if the astigmatism was greater than the sphere, or the elliptical module if the astigmatism was less than or equal to the sphere. In 368 astigmatic eyes, the sequential program was used in 123 eyes (mean astigmatism 2.25 D) and the elliptical module in 245 eyes (mean astigmatism 1.35 D). Attempted correction was between -0.50 D and -6.00

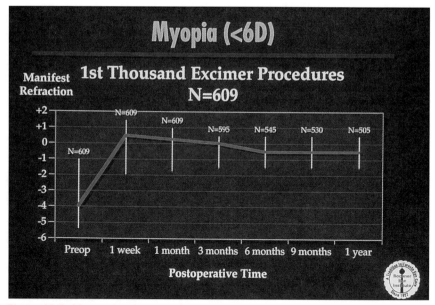

Figure 10-7. Mean refraction over time.

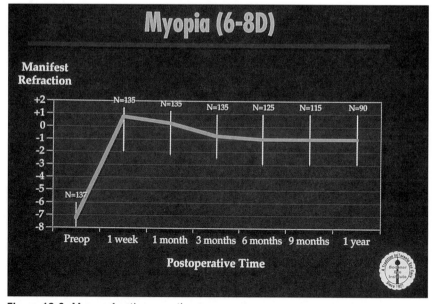

Figure 10-8. Mean refraction over time.

D of myopic astigmatism for both groups. The percentage of astigmatism corrected was 65% for the sequential mode and 85% for the elliptical module. Given the disparity between attempted and achieved correction, the nomogram has been changed to achieve higher levels of correction. Follow-up data with an average follow-up of 18 months reflect the improvement in

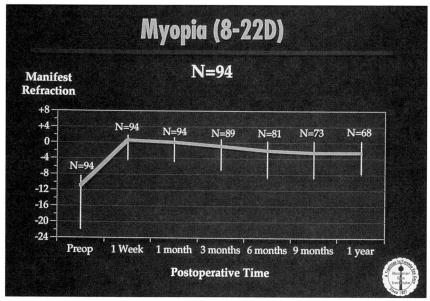

Figure 10-9. Mean refraction over time.

achieved vision.

In all groups, corneal stability based on refraction and videokeratography occurred in 70% by 3 months, 90% by 6 months, and 99% by 12 months. It can be difficult to differentiate between regression and progression of myopia. Generally, the lower the refractive error, the earlier the corneal stability. However, regression was seen in cases of low myopia as well as high myopia.

Overall, at the Bochner Eye Institute and the Beacon Eye Institute, patient satisfaction level has been higher with PRK than with any other ophthalmic surgical procedure. In a questionnaire that was completed by 250 consecutive patients with at least a 1-year follow-up, 92% rated their satisfaction level as being extremely high. Ninety-seven percent of the patients said they would recommend the procedure to a friend or family member. The main factors for satisfaction are the ability to have good uncorrected vision both day and night and an absence of glare or halos.

Loss or Gain of Best-Corrected Acuity

Our studies showed that best spectacle-corrected visual acuity was not reduced by PRK in 98.6% of eyes with a 2-year follow-up. One percent of eyes lost one or more lines of acuity, but 1% gained one or more lines of best-corrected acuity. It is thought that the improvement in acuity is secondary to increased magnification. The decrease in best-corrected visual acuity noted in 1.4% of patients was secondary to central islands, corneal haze, or decentration of the ablation zone. Secondary treatment for their complication has generally been successful in improving the visual outcome.

Symptoms

A small percentage of subjective symptoms were reported during the 2-year period after PRK; decreased night vision was the most common. Other symptoms were decreased quality of vision, halos, and near vision disturbance. Two years after PRK, few patients reported marked symptoms. Of those patients with subjective symptoms, most were satisfied with their visual outcome after PRK.

Refraction

The preoperative average manifest refraction was -5.00 D ±1.21 D. One year postoperatively the mean was -0.45 D ±0.88 D and 0.48 D ±0.89 2 years postoperatively. The maximum hyperopic shift occurred at 1 week and any regression generally stabilized by 6 to 12 months. There was no significant change in pre- and postoperative refractive cylinder at 1 and 2 years postoperatively.

Haze

In most of the patients, a faint diffuse subepithelial haze appeared after 1 month, increasing in intensity during the next 2 to 3 months, and then gradually decreasing. After 2 years, 4.4% had corneal haze of grade 1 that was generally not visually significant. One patient developed a dense central corneal haze that reduced best-corrected visual acuity to 20/60 6 months postoperatively despite the use of topical steroids. He was retreated with an improvement to 20/25 in the early postoperative period, but again developed a significant corneal haze at 6 months that limited his acuity to 20/80. By 2 years postoperatively, his best-corrected acuity improved to 20/25. It was discovered that this patient was a keloid former with multiple prominent scars on his skin. We feel that this is a contraindication to photorefrative surgery. In the future, with the development of additional wound modulating agents, this problem will probably be overcome.

Discussion

Data at our institute and internationally have shown that PRK is a safe procedure, with excellent predictability especially in the lower myopic ranges, and that the results are generally stable after 6 to 12 months. Clinical results in terms of uncorrected and best-corrected visual acuity have improved over time with a better understanding of pre- and postoperative concerns, advances in laser technology, and improvements in surgical techniques. The techniques of multipass and multizone have resulted in less haze and regression. This approach has been adopted by most users of broad beam lasers (ie, VisX, Summit Technology). Experienced laser users seem to achieve excellent results with a wide variety of epithelial removal techniques. Will new lasers that use a slit scanning beam or a small flying spot beam lead to improved visual results with a lower incidence of complications? There is a trend around the world to decrease the frequency and duration of steroid drops postoperatively. Will we continue to use steroid drops in the treatment of higher degrees of myopia? Although the technology is evolving, the worldwide clinical results demonstrate the safety of PRK and the high level of patient satisfaction.

Chapter 11

Role in Astigmatism

By controlling the size, shape, and energy of the laser beam, the surgeon can sculpt the cornea into various shapes. Excimer laser PRK can produce radially symmetric ablations to correct myopic or hyperopic refractive errors and toric ablations to correct astigmatism. McDonnell was the first to create toric ablations, first on plastic spheres, then on rabbit corneas, and finally on human eyes.

Technical Operation

The astigmatism correction with the VisX 20/20 B or STAR laser can be performed either in an elliptical module or a sequential module. It is preferable to use the elliptical module, but one is restricted to cases in which the sphere is greater than or equal to the astigmatism. If the astigmatism is greater than the sphere, the sequential mode is used in which the astigmatism is treated first, then the sphere. With the elliptical module, both the astigmatism and the sphere are treated at the same time, which can achieve better astigmatic results.

Initial work with the VisX 20/20 B excimer laser was to produce corneal transverse excisions to correct astigmatism. The placement and depth of the excision was dependent upon the location of the axis of astigmatism and the degree of correction required. For this procedure a contact mask was required (Figure 11-1A). The excisions could be linear, concave, or convex (Figure 11-1B). All excisions were made perpendicular to the steepest meridian of astigmatism. Unfortunately, there was no advantage of this technique over the use of a diamond blade.

To correct myopia, the VisX excimer laser uses a computer-controlled iris

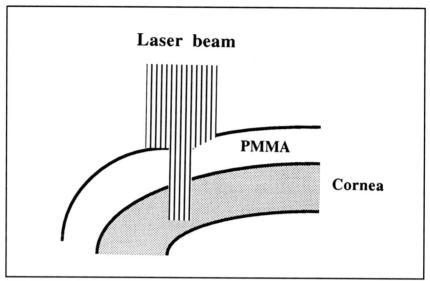

Figure 11-1A. Technique developed initially for treating astigmatism with a mask made of PMMA. Opening in the plastic allowed for excision of tissue.

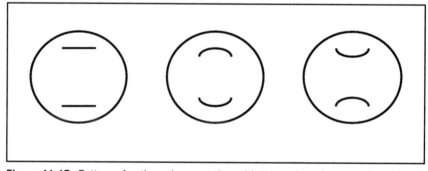

Figure 11-1B. Pattern of astigmatic correction with the excimer laser produced by an overlying mask. There was no advantage of this technique over an AK produced by a diamond blade.

diaphragm to vary the diameter of the circular ablation beam to ablate more tissue centrally than peripherally. To treat myopic astigmatism, the same large-diameter excimer beam is passed through a set of parallel rectangular blades (Figure 11-2). Initially, these blades are closed. As the treatment is carried out, the blades open, flattening the steeper axis of the cornea. The cornea should be flattened only in the meridian perpendicular to the long axis of the slit, termed the mechanical axis. No refractive change is intended along this mechanical axis (long axis of the slit). For example, when the mechanical axis is oriented in the 180° meridian, a flattening of the cornea occurs 90° away from that, in the 90° meridian, with no change in the 180°

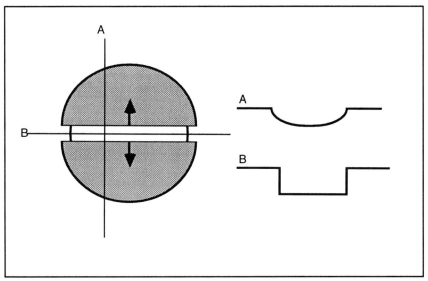

Figure 11-2. The treatment of astigmatism is accomplished by a slit that gradually opens. (A) In the direction of opening of the slit a refractive change occurs. (B) In the opposite meridian there is no significant refractive change.

meridian. The laser can be programmed to treat as low as -0.25 D of astigmatism.

Indications

Congenital Myopic Astigmatism

Naturally occurring myopic astigmatism is usually regular astigmatism with symmetrical steepening in the two steepest hemimeridians. The cornea should be evaluated using videokeratography preoperatively to rule out asymmetric or irregular astigmatism.

Postoperative Astigmatism

After cataract extraction, penetrating keratoplasty (PK), refractive surgical procedures, and post-corneal penetrating trauma, astigmatism can be a major problem limiting visual recovery. Conventional surgery for astigmatism usually involves incisional procedures, including relaxing incisions (radial, transverse, and arcuate), trapezoidal astigmatic keratotomy ([AK] Ruiz procedure), and wedge resection.

Surgical Technique

To correct the cylindrical component of the refraction, we have to take into consideration the best manifest refraction and the corneal topography. The best visual results are obtained when the refractive astigmatic axis is close to the topographic astigmatic axis. In this situation, a spherical cornea results after astigmatic surgery. Unfortunately, in the majority of cases there is often a difference between these two measurements of astigmatism. Stephen Trokel feels that if the astigmatic axis can be moved closer to the topographic axis preoperatively (provided that visual acuity is not significantly affected), the visual outcome can be improved.

After epithelial removal and pretreatment to prevent central islands (see Chapter 8), the astigmatism can be treated by either the sequential or elliptical method as previously discussed. The sequential method is chosen when the cylinder exceeds the spherical component of the refraction. In the sequential method, the amount of minus sphere to be treated is calculated by first determining the expected hyperopic shift. This is calculated by dividing the intended cylinder correction by eight. This amount of expected hyperopic shift is then subtracted from the spherical component to give the intended spherical correction. The cylindrical correction is done first, followed by the spherical correction. The sequential cylindrical ablations are 6.0 mm in the largest dimension, by 5.0 or 4.5 mm in the smallest. The elliptical ablation for the correction of compound myopic astigmatism can be used to correct cylinder and sphere simultaneously. The algorithm produces an ellipse that has no transition zones.

The elliptical ablations are chosen for most cases, providing the cylinder does not exceed the spherical component. In the elliptical method, the cylinder is also corrected first, followed by the myopic spherical correction. The central beam begins as a slit which expands to a 6.0-mm length and then collapses as an ellipse to correct the myopic portion of the treatment. The elliptical ablations are 6.00 mm in the largest dimension and 4.50 mm in the smallest.

Postoperative Management

The postoperative management is the same as discussed in Chapter 9. Computerized videokeratography analysis is helpful in evaluating the centration of the ablation and the overall correction of the cylinder. The difference map, which is obtained by subtracting the preoperative from the postoperative map, is equal to the profile of the ablated corneal tissue.

Future

The excimer laser is not specifically designed to correct irregular or asymmetric astigmatism. Dr. Mihai Pop of Quebec suggests decentering the treatment zone in patients with asymmetric astigmatism, "so even if you take a perfect central laser beam, and you center it on an irregular cornea, you'll have more irregularity after the treatment. I often decenter without losing fixation up to 1.5 to 2 mm." If Pop is treating a patient with 4 D of astigmatism, he will do the first 1 D of correction at the center, then begin to move the beam, without holding the eye.

In patients with irregular astigmatism, it is possible to perform a spherical ablation over the steepest areas of the cornea. After healing has occurred, if the topography is more spherical, a central myopic ablation can be performed. Dr. Don Johnson from Vancouver has used this technique to treat patients with keratoconus.

We conclude that PRK may be useful for treating different types of astigmatism. To evaluate the efficacy and safety of this technique in irregular and asymmetric astigmatism, more studies are necessary. In the future, excimer laser technology will probably be linked to computerized videokeratography data so that any irregular corneal surface can be made spherical or aspheric.

Chapter 12

Hyperopic Photorefractive Keratectomy

A variety of surgical techniques have been developed to correct hyperopia. Non-excimer techniques were developed nearly 100 years ago. Lans was the first to report that heating of the cornea could induce collagen shrinkage with resultant corneal curvature changes. Various collagen shrinkage procedures have evolved since then. Over the years, steepening the cornea by collagen shrinkage has involved the hot needle technique developed by Fyodorov in performing a radial thermokeratoplasty to the use of the holmium:YAG laser.

Hyperopia corrections by noncontact holmium:YAG laser has been reported in several papers over the past few years and remains controversial. Koch et al reported the results in May 1996 in 17 patients for correction up to 3 D. Treatment parameters included simultaneous delivery of eight holmium:YAG laser spots in a symmetrical octagonal array with a centerline diameter of 6 mm, 10 pulses of laser light at 5 Hz pulse repetition frequency, and pulse energies of 159 to 199 mJ. Follow-up was 2 years in 15 of 17 patients. The mean change in spherical equivalent was -0.79 D. Eleven of these 15 eyes (73%) had a mean refractive correction of -1.1 D (range: -0.38 D to -2.63 D). None of the eyes lost two or more lines of spectacle-corrected distance vision. The amount of refractive correction at 2 years after surgery was correlated to the treatment pulse energy and the volume of the opacified corneal tissue observed immediately after treatment. Koch et al concluded that the technique of noncontact LTK produced safe, effective, and persistent correlations of low hyperopia in the majority of treated eyes.

We used the noncontact holmium:YAG laser prior to our current use of

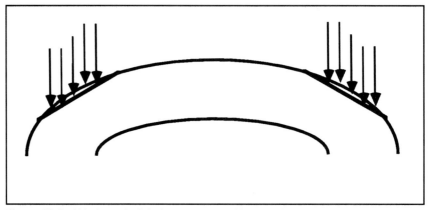

Figure 12-1. Ablation principle for treatment of hyperopia.

the excimer laser in treating hyperopia. There was a definite curvature change and refractive improvement in all patients in the early postoperative period. Unfortunately, the high incidence of regression and corneal instability noted after a few months caused us to abandon this form of hyperopic treatment.

Excimer laser PRK for hyperopia is employed to steepen the anterior cornea. The principle is that the greatest depth of ablation occurs in the mid-periphery with minimal ablation centrally (Figure 12-1).

VisX STAR Laser

Studies have been done to determine the safety and efficacy of excimer PRK for treating hyperopia. The VisX FDA-monitored hyperopic PRK study phase I included only a handful of patients whose treated eyes were legally blind. This study was done by Marguerite B. McDonald of New Orleans. Ten legally blind eyes were treated. The preliminary conclusion of this study was that excimer laser PRK for hyperopia appears to be safe and effective for treating hyperopia.

The VisX STAR corrects hyperopia by a scanning mechanism that spares the central 0.8 mm and treats with an effective optical zone of 5 mm extending the treatment to 9 mm. Jackson from the University of Ottawa has reported on 25 eyes followed for a minimum of 6 months. Average preoperative refractive error was +2.48 D (range: +1.00 D to +4.00 D). At 6 months, the average spherical equivalent was +0.27 D with a standard deviation of ±0.55. At 6 months, uncorrected visual acuity was 20/25 or better in 80%, and 20/40 or better in 88%. Eighty percent of the eyes were within ±0.50 D. Recent communication indicates continued refractive stability at 14 months. The corneas have remained essentially clear with a maximum of trace haze noted.

The VisX STAR has been used by one of us (RMS) to correct overcorrected PRKs. The results in six eyes with a 6-month follow-up have been impressive. Average preoperative spheroequivalent was +1.5 D (range: +1.00 D to +4.25 D). Average postoperative spheroequivalent was -0.27 D with a standard deviation of ±0.55. The corneas that were clear preoperatively were clear postoperatively. There was no increase in haze in corneas that showed preoperative haze. These excellent results indicate that induced hyperopia after myopic PRK can be successfully managed.

Hyperopic PRK with the Aesculap-Meditec MEL-60 excimer laser has been done in Germany and Italy for about 7 years. In a study by Dieter Dausch in Amberg using this laser, four partially sighted and 19 normally sighted hyperopic eyes were treated. Two groups of patients were studied. In the first group of 15 patients, the preoperative refraction ranged from +2.0 D to +7.5 D. In the second group of eight aphakic patients, the preoperative refraction ranged from +11 D to +16 D.

The diameter of the corrected zone was 4 mm, the overall diameter was 7 mm, and there was a 1.5-mm transition zone ring on all sides. A mask with a spiral aperture was used with the Aesculap-Meditec laser. This aperture had to be turned by a fixed angle (eg, 4°) between individual laser exposures. The ablation process was completed when the total rotation reached 360°. The mask had to be inserted into a suction ring, which was first adjusted and fixed to the patient's eye. The operation mask must be situated exactly in the optical center of the cornea.

Preoperatively, the mean corrected visual acuity of group I (+2.00 D to +7.50 D) was 20/25, ranging from 20/100 to 20/20. Postoperatively the mean was 20/30, ranging from 20/100 to 20/20. In group II (+11.00 D to +16.00 D), the mean preoperative corrected acuity was 20/35, ranging from 20/50 to 20/22, decreasing postoperatively to a mean of 20/57 (range 20/100 to 20/40).

Mean preoperative visual acuity under glare was 20/40 in group I and 20/100 in group II. At 12 months, glare visual acuity was 20/50 in group I and <20/200 in group II.

One month following surgery a subepithelial ring of haze was detectable in all eyes. The mean haze in group I was 1.25 and in group II was 2.0. The haze intensity increased over the following 2 months, and gradually decreased to 0.8 in group I and 2.1 in group II. The refraction mean postoperative in group I was +1.0 D and in group II was +3.0 D.

In this study the regression (loss of effect) was more marked in the eyes with higher corrections. Correction of higher hyperopia with excimer laser requires a deeper stromal ablation and a more abrupt change in curvature at the edge of the ablation. The percentage of treated eyes within ±1.0 D of emmetropia was 80% in group I and 37% in group II.

The haze after PRK for hyperopia with the Meditec laser has a ring shape, while the center of the cornea remains clear. For this reason the haze intensity after PRK for hyperopia does not affect visual acuity. It is believed that the loss of best-corrected visual acuity in hyperope is due to a decentration of the ablated zone by more than 1 mm from the center of the cornea. In fact, the videokeratography showed the decentration to be greatest (1.0 to 1.3 mm) in eyes with a loss of corrected vision.

Halo and glare problems are most intense immediately after surgery. After 12 months these subjective symptoms were more important in group II.

Another study was carried out by Till Anschutz in Germany, with the Aesculap-Meditec excimer laser. The ablation zone was first marked with a centration marker consisting of two concentric rings. A rotating hyperopic spiral mask with an optical zone of 4 mm and an ablation zone of 7 mm was used. The rotating spiral mask creates a steepening of the cornea with a peripheral furrow.

This study was divided into three groups: group I had 34 patients with 2.00 D to 5.00 D of hyperopia, group II had 17 patients with 5.25 D to 10.00 D, and group III (aphakic) ranged from 10.25 D to 15.00 D, with a follow-up of 2 years.

The best results were in group I. In this group the mean reduction of hyperopia was 3.5 D and the mean regression was 1.5 D. In group II, the mean regression was 3.5 D, and in group III Anschutz found that PRK could not reduce hyperopia more than 7 D or 8 D. The predictability was 70% in group I and 38% in group II. Anschutz believes that the biggest problems with the excimer laser surgery for hyperopia are the small optical zone and centration procedure.

Nidek EC-5000 Laser

Alignment

We have been using the Nidek EC-5000 primarily for hyperopia. We have had to modify the nomogram a number of times to result in an effective correction. Our technique is somewhat the same as for myopia but we use a 9.0 mm removal of the epithelium.

Epithelial Removal Technique at 9.0-mm Diameter

- Mechanical with 9.0-mm zone
- Alcohol or brush with 9.0-mm zone

The relevant data and the prescription of the patient are entered. The treatment zone is 5.5 mm and the transition zone is 9.0 mm for hyperopia.

The laser is ready to ablate. A minimal amount of tissue is ablated from the center of the cornea and deeper ablation is achieved in the periphery according to the patient prescription.

Results

We have only been using the Nidek for 1 year for hyperope at the time of this writing. The immediate results have been impressive. We have tried two aphakes with 10 D prescription who were scheduled for secondary IOL implantation. Early results were impressive for hyperope for these patients. We have similar early results with lower hyperope and astigmatism. It is still to early to draw any conclusions as the majority of ablations for hyperopia are in the past 6 months.

Summary

With these results we conclude that PRK for hyperopia is a promising modality. As in PRK for myopia, accurate centration of the procedure is one component of the technique that is critical to its success. Also, larger optical zones and large ablation zones are necessary to improve the results.

Phototherapeutic Keratectomy

PTK with the excimer laser has been shown to be an effective treatment for many anterior corneal pathologies, to remove superficial opacities, and to smooth the anterior corneal surface.

On March 21, 1994, the US FDA-approved Summit Technology and VisX to sell their ArF 193-nm excimer lasers for the treatment of superficial corneal scars, opacities, and irregularities.

The excimer laser for therapeutic use offers tremendous potential for improving sight to literally millions of individuals affected by corneal scars, dystrophies, or degenerations. Superficial ablation of the stroma up to 150 μm in depth can remove opacities and permit normal regularly aligned stromal fibers to be covered by regenerated epithelial cells.

The use of the excimer in corneal surgery enables surgeons to treat a variety of corneal conditions, obviating the need of a corneal transplant (Figure 13-1). Unlike a corneal transplant, with a PTK there is no risk of endophthalmitis, graft rejection, or suture breakage. In addition, the recovery period is relatively rapid, with the majority of patients seeing reasonably well in a few weeks. Successful PTK depends on a thorough preoperative assessment and attention to detail when performing the procedure.

Contraindications

Contraindications to PTK include:
- Keratoconus with corneal thickness <250 μm
- Significant corneal neovascularization in the ablation zone that cannot be occluded with either electrocautery or the argon laser

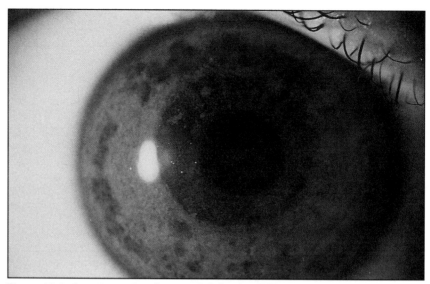

Figure 13-1. A postoperative photograph following PTK for superficial variant of granular dystrophy. Best-corrected visual acuity improved from 20/200 to 20/50.

- Scars deeper than 150 μm
- Advanced keratitis sicca with superficial punctate keratopathy or corneal filaments

Preoperative Evaluation

It is very important during a preoperative evaluation to rule out the factors that are contraindications for PTK, and evaluate the type and depth of pathology. Different types of pathology ablate at different rates. For example, it is much easier and faster to ablate the corneal stroma than calcium. Depth of pathology requires a careful evaluation with a slit lamp, and cannot be done with the operating microscope.

Preoperative Concerns

In performing PTK, there are a number of preoperative concerns that may determine the suitability of a given patient. The first concern is that of location of the corneal opacity (Figure 13-2). Ideal cases are those in which the corneal opacity is subepithelial and homogeneous. Elevated nodules of the central cornea can be easily treated with the excimer laser, such as in the case of Salzmann's nodules. Depressed scars are difficult to treat because of the irregular nature of the overlying surface. Deep scars are contraindicated because of the risk of perforation. It is generally felt that opacities in the anterior 150 μm can be treated with the excimer laser.

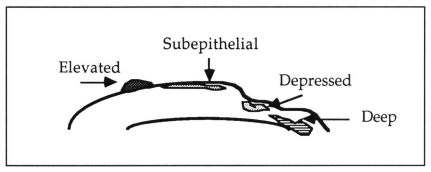

Figure 13-2. Location of corneal opacities.

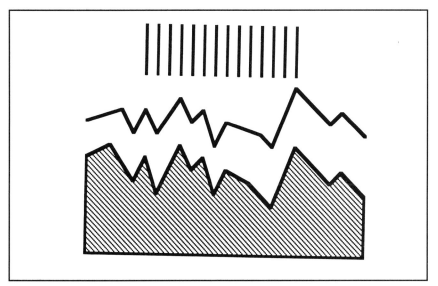

Figure 13-3A. Diagram illustrating an irregular surface preoperatively and postoperatively.

The second preoperative concern is that of the overlying corneal topography. If one has an irregular surface preoperatively, then frequently the postoperative cornea will be irregular (Figures 13-3A and 13-3B). The goal in the treatment of irregular surfaces is to try to fill in the valleys with a masking agent to produce a smoother anterior surface, which in effect will result in a smooth postoperative surface. Masking agents that have been tried with some success include artificial tears, Healon, and Amvisc. It is interesting that the histopathology of stromal scars is often associated with overlying epithelial hyperplasia and thinning that produces a relatively smooth anterior corneal surface (Figure 13-4). In effect, the epithelium acts like a masking agent, and therefore, when a PTK procedure is performed,

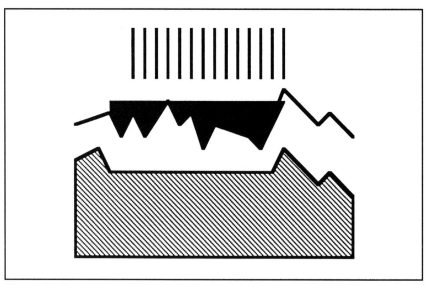

Figure 13-3B. A masking agent can be use to fill in the valleys to create a smoother anterior surface which results in a smoother postoperative surface.

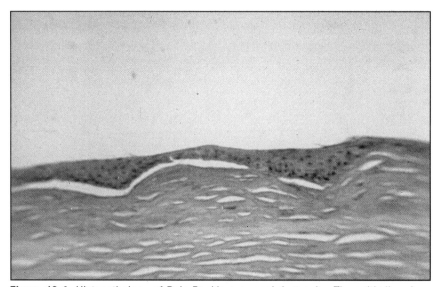

Figure 13-4. Histopathology of Reis-Bucklers corneal dystrophy. The epithelium has undergone hyperplasia or thickening in areas to smooth the anterior corneal surface.

except in cases of anterior basement membrane dystrophy, the laser is used to ablate through the epithelium to reach the stroma, producing superior visual results.

The third concern is that of vascularization (Figure 13-5). If bleeding occurs during the procedure, then the blood can block the laser beam with a

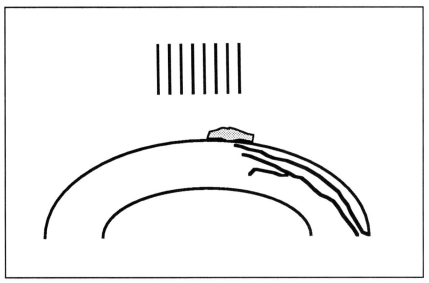

Figure 13-5. A vascularized cornea will bleed during laser surgery and the blood will interfere with the laser ablation.

reduced effect on the cornea. It is important to occlude vessels preoperatively, which in the case of superficial vascularization can be done with a hand-held cautery at the slit lamp, or in the case of deep active vessels with the argon laser.

The fourth preoperative concern is that of refractive error (Figure 13-6). In the majority of cases of PTK there is a hyperopic shift, the severity of which is dependent on the depth of ablation. Ideal cases, therefore, are patients who are myopic with superficial opacities. In these cases the refractive error and the corneal haze can be corrected together. A significant hyperopic shift may induce anisometropia that may necessitate wearing a contact lens. It is also reasonable to perform a hyperopic PRK in the management of hyperopia following PTK.

Indications

Therapeutic areas in which the excimer laser can be useful are:
- Removal of superficial scars and irregularities on the cornea as a result of trauma and infections
- Removal of anterior corneal dystrophies, corneal degenerations, and deposits such as band keratopathy
- Removal of superficial corneal ulcers such as fungal ulcers (to allow for deeper penetration of topical medications)

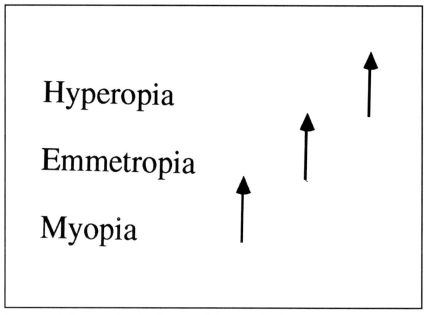

Figure 13-6. The shift in refractive error following a PTK.

- Smoothing of corneal surface after excision of a neoplasm (eg, squamous cell carcinoma)
- Following pterygium surgery

In other words, the excimer laser is useful in removing any opacifications of the superficial layers of the cornea while retaining the health and clarity of the deeper layers.

Recurrent Corneal Erosions

Recurrent corneal erosions occur due to abnormalities in the epithelial basement membrane. There are a variety of etiologies, such as secondary to trauma and anterior basement membrane dystrophy.

The excimer laser breaches Bowman's layer so that the anterior stroma stimulates fibroblast healing and new basement membrane formation. Increasing the number of hemidesmosomes improves adhesion. With scanning electron microscopy at high magnification using eye bank corneas, it appears that the ablated surface has been roughened by the laser. This effect may account for the improved epithelial adhesions.

Corneal Scars and Dystrophy

The category of corneal scars and dystrophy include pathologic conditions such as anterior stromal and superficial leukomas from post-infectious and post-traumatic causes, including inactive herpes simplex virus, keratitis, anterior corneal dystrophies, and Salzmann's degeneration. In addition, the laser can be used to vaporize any residual central scarring following pterygium surgery.

The intraoperative evaluation of the amount of residual scar is important and requires temporary cessation of the laser ablation and slit lamp examination to determine the amount of residual scar after a preprogrammed number of pulses can be delivered.

Deposits

Superficial corneal deposits can be ablated with the excimer laser. The most common deposit is that of calcium or band keratopathy. Since the deposits are located in Bowman's layer, theoretically <20 μm of tissue need to be ablated. The problem, however, is that it is difficult to estimate prior to laser ablation the number of required pulses, since calcium granules can be relatively soft in some cases and extremely hard in others. The harder the granules, the more pulses that are required for a complete ablation. After a set number of pulses, the patient can be taken to the slit lamp to determine central clarity and the necessity of additional treatment.

Corneal Nodule

Frequently patients with keratoconus develop a nodule at the apex of the cone and become unable to wear contact lenses. The goal of PTK is to flatten the nodule so that contact lens use can be resumed.

To flatten the corneal nodule, PTK can usually be done at 2.5-mm diameter. The results can be dramatic, allowing patients to wear contact lenses without discomfort or dislocation.

Microbial Keratitis

UV irradiation of the excimer laser can be used to eliminate microorganisms from the surface of the eye. The problem, however, is that many serious corneal infections are relatively deep, and the use of the laser could lead to a perforation. It is important to realize that microbial keratitis is a medical condition, and the mainstay of treatment is with antimicrobial medication. Although the laser may play a role in refractory cases, it would only be as adjunctive therapy.

Surgical Technique

In performing PTK, the same methods of calibrating the laser machine and performing a list of safety checks are undertaken in a similar manner to that in performing PRK (see Chapter 8). Preoperative medication consists of a nonsteroidal drop, a topical antibiotic, and an anesthetic drop prior to laser

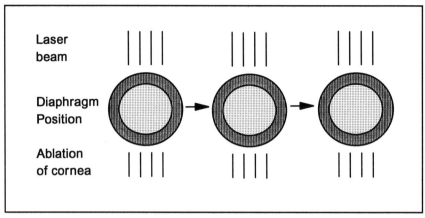

Laser
beam

Diaphragm
Position

Ablation
of cornea

Figure 13-7. Relationship between laser beam, diaphragm, and the laser that makes contact with the cornea. Since the diaphragm stays completely open during the procedure, this minimizes the refractive change.

surgery. The area of ablation may vary in size, usually between 2 and 6 mm.

If the patient is myopic, a PRK may be performed in order to correct the myopia and vaporize the corneal opacity at the same time. The ability of performing PRK in these cases is dependent on the required depth of ablation to remove the corneal haze vs. the depth required to correct the refractive error.

Patients who are emmetropic or hyperopic are usually treated with a PTK mode. In this mode the diaphragm of the laser stays open from beginning to end, minimizing the refractive change (Figure 13-7).

A masking agent, such as an artificial tear (methylcellulose 0.5% to 2%), may be used to fill in the valleys to create a smoother anterior corneal surface prior to corneal ablation. PTK is a dynamic procedure. The surgeon should be prepared to make changes at the surgical plane during the procedure. If the masking agent is dispersed from its intended site, then the procedure is stopped and additional wetting agent is applied to the corneal surface.

Unlike PRK surgery, patients with corneal scars or dystrophies may be taken back to the slit lamp following laser surgery to determine the precise location of any residual opacities. If the opacities are superficial, then additional laser treatment can be applied. Postoperatively, a bandage contact lens is used along with an antibiotic, a steroid drop, and a nonsteroidal medication (see Chapter 9). The nonsteroidal, as in photorefractive surgery, is used for pain control and can often be discontinued after 2 days. The bandage soft contact lens is removed when the epithelium is healed, usually after 2 to 4 days.

Table 13-1.
Postoperative Visual Results in the Treatment
of Scar and Dystrophies

	Number	Improved	Visual Acuity Same	Worse
HSV	18	11	3	4
Epstein-Barr	4	4	0	0
Bacterial	23	15	5	3
Chemical	10	7	2	1
Pterygia	14	10	4	0
Trachoma	20	16	3	1
Dystrophies	27	25	2	0
Total	116	88 (77%)	19 (16%)	9 (7%)

Results

One hundred seventy-five eyes were treated at the Bochner Eye Institute using the VisX 20/20 B laser between October 1991 and January 1996 with an average follow-up of 36 months and a range of 6 to 54 months. Of the 175 cases, 60 were for corneal scars, 15 for corneal dystrophies, 22 for deposits, and 38 for recurrent corneal erosions.

Corneal Scars and Dystrophies

In reviewing our data for corneal scars and dystrophies (Table 13-1), 77% of the patients showed an improvement in visual acuity of two or more lines. Sixteen percent of patients showed no change in visual acuity, and 7% showed a deterioration of acuity of two or more lines. Of the patients who showed an improvement, 80% had 20/40 or better acuity postoperatively. Of the patients who showed a deterioration of visual acuity, the majority have undergone a PK without complications.

Complications that can occur in performing PTK for scars and dystrophies include corneal haze, hyperopic shift, irregular astigmatism, recurrence of a dystrophy, or recurrence of herpes simplex viral keratitis.

Corneal Deposits

Corneal deposits secondary to calcium, as in band keratopathy, can be easily treated with the excimer laser, creating a clear central zone. Since the calcium granules are located in Bowman's layer, the depth of ablation can be limited. It is unlikely that the recurrence of these deposits is any different with laser treatment than with a chelating agent. There is less induced inflammation with the excimer laser than with other surgical alternatives.

Recurrent Corneal Erosions

At the Bochner Eye Institute, we treated 38 eyes with recurrent corneal erosions in 27 patients. Sixty percent of these eyes had anterior membrane dystrophy, and 40% were secondary to a traumatic injury. These 38 eyes were refractory to hypertonic drops and ointment in all cases, a bandage contact lens in 14 eyes, epithelial debridement in six eyes, and anterior stromal micropuncture in six eyes.

The PTK technique was to debride the epithelium mechanically. Since the epithelium in anterior basement membrane dystrophy is often irregular, it is best not to perform a transepithelial approach, as there is a risk of inducing irregular astigmatism. The epithelium is easily removed. The depth of stromal ablation was limited to 5 to 10 μm. If the erosions were recurring in a central location, a 6-mm optical zone, then an eccentric ablation of 2 to 3 mm was performed. As in PRK, the patients were fit with a soft contact lens and were to use a nonsteroidal drop along with an antibiotic and a topical steroid.

Our results showed that 34 of 38 eyes (89%) were without a recurrence following laser surgery, with an average follow-up of 28 months and a range of 6 to 51 months. The average shift in refractive error was +0.25 D to +0.50 D.

It appears that recurrent corneal erosions can be successfully treated by the excimer laser. In all probability, the recurrence of erosions will increase with the duration of the follow-up. It appears that patients who recur, and who are again refractory to routine medical measures, can be retreated with the excimer laser.

Problems

Some of the inherent problems in performing a PTK include:

- The ablation rates can differ for calcium deposits, scars, and the normal stroma. Because of this irregular ablation pattern, an irregular surface may be produced, necessitating the wearing of a rigid gas-permeable lens for optimum acuity.
- The masking agents that are used today are not ideal. A perfect masking agent would be stable during the procedure and not be dispersed by the laser beam. The masking agent would ablate at the same rate as the corneal stroma. The anterior surface of the masking agent should be smooth to create a smooth postoperative surface.

Summary

In conclusion, PTK offers real clinical benefits to patients with corneal scars, dystrophies, deposits, and recurrent corneal erosions. Patient selection is critical in achieving satisfactory results. The procedure is generally more difficult to perform than PRK, as there are no nomograms to determine how much tissue to remove.

At the Bochner Eye Institute, we have found that PTK may be an alternative to PK surgery in approximately 10% to 15% of referred patients. Although the results are encouraging, there will continue to be improvements in the future with the development of superior masking agents, and flying spot excimer technology that can be guided by computerized videokeratography.

Complications

Chapter 14

Potential Complications and Management Guidelines

C linicians must understand and recognize the potential complications of PRK. With an appreciation of the possible complications, prophylactic precautions can often be taken to minimize the development of these complications. In addition, the eyecare practitioner who recognizes the early symptoms and signs of these complications can initiate appropriate treatment and/or reassure the patient. In this section, potential complications and guidelines for treatment are discussed.

Complications can be divided into the following categories:

A. Possible Side Effects of Corticosteroid Use
   1. Ocular Hypertension
B. Early (<6 weeks) Complications
   1. Discomfort/Pain
   2. Corneal Infection/Sterile Infiltrates
   3. Delayed Epithelial Healing
   4. Pseudodendrites
C. Early and/or Late Complications
   1. Loss of Best-Corrected Visual Acuity
   2. Halo Effect
   3. Central Islands
   4. Decentration
   5. Recurrent Corneal Erosion
D. Late (>6 weeks) Complications
   1. Diffuse Haze
   2. Arcuate or Peripheral Haze

E. Refractive Complications
1. Undercorrection
2. Overcorrection
3. Presbyopia
4. Regression With or Without Haze
F. General Awareness
1. Pregnancy
2. Eye Sensitivity

Possible Side Effects of Corticosteroid Use

Ocular Hypertension

Clinical Features

In a small percentage of patients, the postoperative use of steroids can result in increased IOP. Reduction or discontinuation of the steroid dose and application of beta blockers typically return the IOP to normal.

It is critical that you monitor IOP following the excimer procedure while the patient continues to use topical steroids.

To reduce the incidence of such occurrence, FML has become the postoperative topical steroid of choice, compared to a more penetrating steroid such as prednisolone acetate or dexamethasone.

Other potential complications associated with the use of topical steroids include:

- Reactivation of latent herpes simples virus which can be treated with antiviral medications.
- Ptosis with an effect on muscle tissue. This tends to occur more often in young women.
- Posterior subcapsular cataracts induced by the chronic, frequent use of steroid drops.

Management

With an elevation in IOP (>23 mmHg), add a beta blocker (if there are no contraindications: asthma, heart block) and recheck IOP. Follow closely and if not improved, taper off FML drops. Reduce frequency until IOP is controlled. Other complications resulting from the use of topical steroids are typically addressed by discontinuing steroid use.

Early (<6 weeks) Complications

Discomfort/Pain

Clinical Features

Patients may experience postoperative discomfort that is similar to that of a corneal abrasion. Ninety percent of patients report little to no discomfort after the PRK and 10% of patients report discomfort or pain which is usually resolved in 24 to 36 hours following the procedure. Most patients today who have discomfort describe it as the sensation of having sand or an eyelash in their eye.

Management

The postoperative pain has been greatly reduced or eliminated by the use of nonsteroidal anti-inflammatory drugs (eg, ketorolac tromethamine 0.5% [Acular] or diclofenac sodium 0.1% [Voltaren]) during the first few days following the PRK procedure in combination with a bandage soft contact lens. It is thought that the pain reduction or elimination is related to the effect of nonsteroidal anti-inflammatory drugs on inhibiting prostaglandin synthesis. By irrigating the eye with balanced saline solution at the completion of the PRK procedure, this decreases the chances of trapped epithelial debris under the bandage lens. This epithelial debris is a source of discomfort in the postoperative period. Systemic medication (eg, Demerol, Tylenol #3) may be used if necessary. Cold compresses applied to the lids are often helpful. In patients with a dry eye, the wearing of a soft contact lens during the first few days after the PRK procedure can result in some irritation or discomfort. This discomfort can often be relieved by the frequent use of artificial tears. Preservative-free brands are recommended. Dry eye patients may benefit from the insertion of collagen implants into the puncta to increase the tear meniscus.

Corneal Infection/Sterile Infiltrates

Clinical Features

Symptoms

Occasionally patients are asymptomatic early in the course. Pain, discharge, or redness may be present (Figure 14-1).

Signs

A corneal infection usually involves a single white infiltrate and an associated purulent discharge. Sterile infiltrates are frequently multiple in

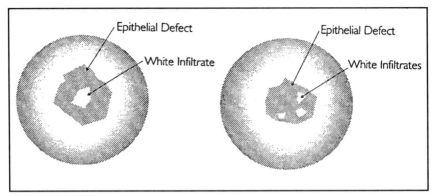

Figure 14-1. Corneal ulcer vs. sterile infiltrates. Courtesy of Beacon Eye Institute.

number without an associated discharge.

Management

Corneal infection and/or sterile infiltrates are rare complications and have been reported to occur, on average, in one out of every 500 cases. These corneal problems are usually recognized on the second to fourth postoperative day. To treat the complication, remove the soft contact lens and send it for bacterial culture and drug sensitivities. A corneal scraping is also recommended for culture and drug sensitivities. Treat as a bacterial corneal ulcer with broad spectrum antibiotics. If the white infiltrate is small, <2 mm in size, consider the use of Ocuflox or Ciloxan every hour during the day and taper with an improvement in the clinical course. If the infiltrate is >2 mm, consider treating with fortified antibiotics, for example, tobramycin 15 mg/cc and cefazolin 50 mg/cc every 30 to 60 minutes and gradually taper. If there is no purulent discharge, and there are multiple infiltrates, consider cautiously adding a topical steroid to counteract a possible immune reaction secondary to the nonsteroidal anti-inflammatory drug.

Delayed Epithelial Healing

Clinical Features

Symptoms
Persistent blurred vision occurs with an epithelial defect (Figure 14-2).

Signs
The epithelial defect usually has well-defined borders. The stroma may show folds secondary to edema.

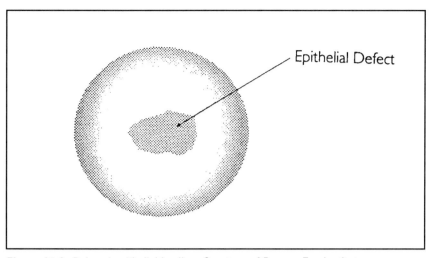

Figure 14-2. Delayed epithelial healing. Courtesy of Beacon Eye Institute.

Management

If the epithelial surface is not intact by 4 days postoperatively, initiate the following steps:

1. Discontinue all drops except the antibiotic. Be sure the patient is not self-medicating with topical anesthetic.
2. If the soft contact lens put in place after the PRK procedure is still present, remove lens and insert a new lens.
3. If the contact lens has been removed, then one may wish to reinsert another protective contact lens.
4. After the epithelium is intact, remove the protective lens and restart the topical steroid.

Pseudodendrites

Clinical Features

Symptoms

Vision may be blurred if the pseudodendrite is in the visual axis (Figure 14-3).

Management

Pseudodendrites are not true complications, but rather a normal healing response. Do not confuse this with a herpetic lesion. A pseudodendritic pattern may be seen as the epithelial surface becomes intact in the healing process during the third and fourth days after the laser procedure. This is a normal healing pattern and will resolve within a few days. No change in the medication is required.

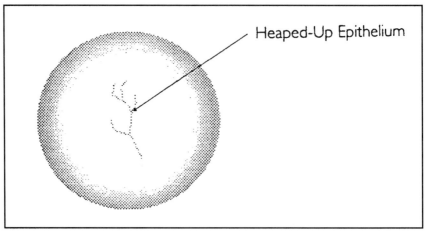

Heaped-Up Epithelium

Figure 14-3. Pseudodendrite represents a normal epithelial healing pattern. Courtesy of Beacon Eye Institute.

Early and/or Late Complications

Loss of Best-Corrected Visual Acuity

Clinical Features

The etiology of blurred vision, or loss of best-corrected visual acuity, can usually be detected with the standard eye examination. Occasionally, computerized videokeratography may be necessary to detect more subtle causes for loss of visual acuity.

Typical causes of loss of best-corrected visual acuity include:
- Epithelial irregularity
- Central islands
- Corneal haze
- Decentered ablation

Vision is typically very blurry immediately after the procedure. It generally starts to improve once the epithelium has grown back, which in most cases takes 2 to 4 days. However, vision can continue to be blurry for a number of weeks. After the epithelial defect has healed, loss of best-corrected visual acuity is usually secondary to an irregular epithelium, which usually smoothes out over a few weeks. Longer term, some patients can lose the ability to read one to two lines of Snellen acuity in comparison to their previous best-corrected vision. With higher corrections, more variability is expected.

Ideal clinical findings are shown in Table 14-1.

Table 14-1
Ideal Clinical Findings

	Uncorrected Visual Acuity	Corneal Haze
Day 10	20/40	trace
Month 1	20/30	trace
Month 2	20/25+	mild
Month 3	20/20	mild
Month 6	20/20	trace
Month 12	20/20	clear

Management

If epithelial irregularity with or without superficial punctate keratitis (SPK) is noted, non-preserved artificial tears should be added. Loss of acuity from other previously listed causes should be managed as outlined in this section. (Refer to appropriate complication section for management guidelines.)

Halo Effect

Clinical Features

Halos may be experienced in the first 4 to 6 weeks following the procedure as the epithelium heals and smoothes out over the complete ablation zone.

Symptoms are more apt to occur at night when dilation of the pupil allows light transmission at the edge of the ablation zone. Persistent halos rarely occur and are usually related to large pupils or a decentered ablation (Figure 14-4).

Management

With most patients, the halo effect tends to diminish with time. In a case that the patient is undercorrected, retreatment with a larger optical zone may alleviate the halos. Halos can also be minimized through the use of pilocarpine drops which constrict the pupil; however, care must be exercised as most patients are intolerant of these drops.

Central Islands

Clinical Features

Central islands, which represent small elevated islands of tissue left centrally, may occur following PRK (Figure 14-5).

Central islands may cause monocular diplopia or blurred vision. The

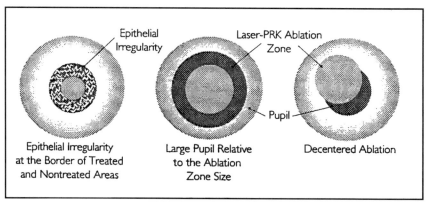

Figure 14-4. Halos may be secondary to epithelial irregularity, a large pupil, or a decentered ablation. Courtesy of Beacon Eye Institute.

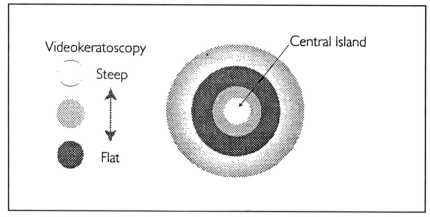

Figure 14-5. Central island represents a central area of steepening. Courtesy of Beacon Eye Institute.

definition of a central island is a central or pericentral area of steepening that is:

- At least 1.00 D in height
- A diameter of at least 1 mm
- Measured at least 1 month postoperatively

    Patients may be asymptomatic or experience qualitative visual changes.

    The islands may be visible as a small central shadow on retinoscopy. The diagnosis can be confirmed with computerized videokeratography showing an elevation within the central or pericentral zone.

    A number of theories have been proposed to explain the cause of central islands.

    Those theories include:

- Vortex plume theory in which the ablated debris interferes with the laser pulses

- Degradation of optics leading to reduced ablation centrally
- Epithelial hyperplasia or thickening which has been documented through use of sophisticated ultrasound techniques
- Acoustic shockwave theory in which each pulse produces a shockwave that leads to stromal hydration
- A theory that the flat and homogeneous laser beam profile produces central fluid accumulation at the time of the procedure which results in decreased ablation centrally

Etiology is probably multifactorial.

Management

The prevention of central islands can be achieved by producing additional pulses to the central cornea. With the VisX laser, a pretreatment of 1 µm/D to the central 2.5 mm has been useful in preventing islands for patients under -6.00 D. For higher degrees of myopia with multizone techniques, 0.6 µm/D is sufficient.

If central islands are noted, the majority of these islands disappear after a period of months. If after 10 months there is a persistent symptomatic central island, the laser can be used to vaporize the central elevation.

Decentration

Clinical Features

Decentration can occur if the laser beam is not precisely aligned with the surgeon's eyepiece prior to the procedure. Poor patient fixation can also cause decentration (Figure 14-6).

Significant eye movement on the part of the patient when the laser is pulsing can create decentration; however, the ophthalmologist has the ability to stop the laser procedure at any point to prevent this potential problem. A small amount of eye movement will typically not affect the outcome of the procedure.

Management

Although a number of approaches have been used to treat the effects of decentration, none at present is completely satisfactory.

Recurrent Corneal Erosion

Clinical Features

Symptoms

Patients may complain of pain, tearing, and photophobia. This is more

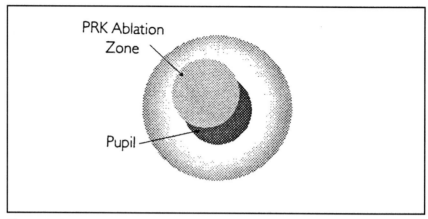

Figure 14-6. Decentered ablation. Courtesy of Beacon Eye Institute.

common in the morning upon awakening. The symptoms may resolve in an hour or persist for hours, if significant (Figure 14-7).

Signs
An epithelial defect or erosion may be seen during the acute episode. Epithelial microcysts may be noted after the erosion has healed.

Management
Recurrent corneal erosions are more common with mechanical epithelial debridement than with laser transepithelial removal. The erosion tends to occur outside the laser area of ablation. Management is similar to that of a recurrent corneal erosion with hypertonic drops and ointment. If this is not satisfactory in preventing a recurrence, a soft contact lens can be tried. If this is not successful, a PTK can be performed to the eroding area. The epithelium in the area is gently removed and a PTK with an optical zone of 2 to 6 mm to encompass the erosion site is selected with a depth of 5 to 8 μm.

Late (>6 weeks) Complications

Diffuse Haze

Clinical Features
Corneal haze usually takes the form of a fine reticular subepithelial pattern that does not interfere with vision. Corneal clarity is graded on a scale of 0 to 4+. The haze corresponds to a corneal healing response following PRK induced by activation and migration of keratocytes (fibroblasts) and newly

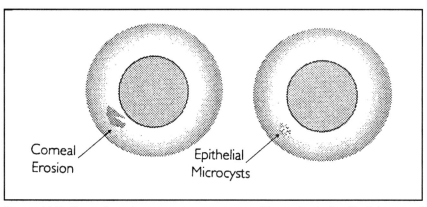

Figure 14-7. Corneal erosions are more common with mechanical epithelial removal outside of the laser treatment zone. Courtesy of Beacon Eye Institute.

synthesized collagen. Results of our first 1000 cases at the Bochner Eye Institute are represented in Figures 14-8 through 14-10. The haze is first noted between 2 and 4 months. The haze gradually fades away by 6 to 12 months. Severe haze rarely occurs. There are some factors that may be related to increased haze: depth of ablation, laser beam homogeneity, epithelial removal method, corneal dryness during treatment, keratitis sicca, solar exposure, and keloid formation. Age does not seem to be an enhancing factor (Figure 14-11).

Management

If the patient has moderate or severe haze that interferes with vision, steroid drops should be increased in frequency to five times per day and gradually tapered over 2 to 3 months. Topical steroids are used to try to modulate the stromal wound healing response. The mechanism is decreased DNA synthesis, as well as lens specific anti-anabolic effects, leading to decreased keratocyte activity and decreased collagen synthesis. Rarely, a persistent haze can occur that may require a repeat laser treatment. It is usually best to treat the haze with a no-touch technique using a PTK mode. Any residual refractive error can be managed in the future with a PRK. The refractive error tends not to be reliable when there is sufficient corneal haze. In about 80% of these cases there is no recurrence of the haze following treatment.

Arcuate or Peripheral Haze

Clinical Features

Haze in the peripheral area of the ablation bed can lead to a hyperopic shift and/or induced astigmatism (Figure 14-12).

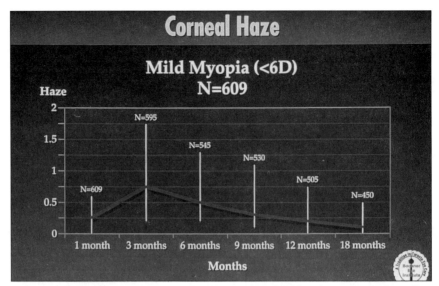

Figure 14-8. Mean haze score over time in a series of PRK cases at the Bochner Eye Institute having <6 D of myopia preoperatively.

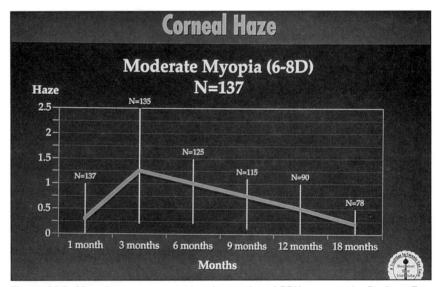

Figure 14-9. Mean haze score over time in a series of PRK cases at the Bochner Eye Institute having 6 D to 8 D of myopia preoperatively.

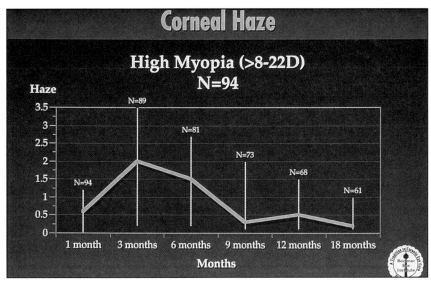

Figure 14-10. Mean haze score over time in a series of PRK cases at the Bochner Eye Institute having >8 D to 22 D of myopia preoperatively.

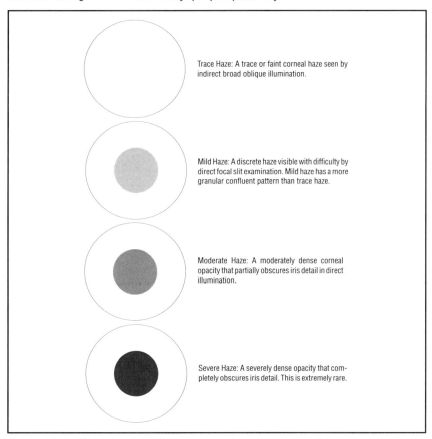

Figure 14-11. Haze classifications.

This peripheral haze is more commonly seen with a laser epithelial ablation. In this case, a steep transition between the ablation zone and the untreated area exists in the periphery of the ablation, where the depth of penetration is most pronounced.

Management

Peripheral haze should be managed as in the case of diffuse haze with the frequent use of steroid drops five times per day with a gradual tapering over 2 to 3 months. This is the only situation in which steroid drops are increased when dealing with a hyperopic refractive error.

Refractive Complications

Undercorrection

Clinical Features

Patients complain of blurred distance vision. The residual myopia is due to insufficient initial treatment which is more common with higher degrees of myopia. Undercorrection may result from an excessively moist cornea during the procedure.

Management

No change from the routine drop protocol is required. If there is an undercorrection and the patient is not satisfied with the level of vision and is not interested in monovision, additional treatment can be performed. It is usually best to wait until the refraction is stable, typically a minimum of 6 months following the initial PRK vision correction procedure.

Overcorrection

Clinical Features

Patients may experience blurred vision when viewing close-up objects. In some cases, particularly with those patients over 40 who are presbyopic, vision may also be blurry when viewing objects in the distance. A small amount of initial overcorrection is acceptable since some regression will often take place. Possible causes include a cornea that is too dry during the procedure and manifest preoperative refraction that did not account for accommodation.

Management

Any significant degree of hyperopia should be managed by tapering the

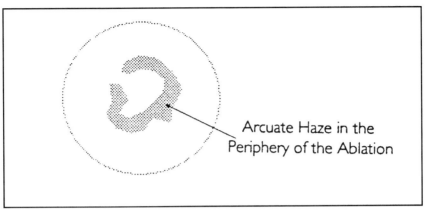

Figure 14-12. Arcuate haze. Courtesy of Beacon Eye Institute.

Table 14-2	
Preoperative Refractive Error	**If Hyperopia is ⩾ Than Below**
1 D and 6 D	+1.25 D
>6 D and <10 D	+1.75 D
10 D and 15 D	+2.25 D

steroid drops over 2 weeks, for example, two times a day for 1 week then QD for 1 week. A more rapid withdrawal of steroids can lead to significant haze. If regression toward myopia is not satisfactory, then epithelial debridement can promote an inflammatory response leading to regression.

If the patient's regression is close to a plano prescription, then drops should be restarted to prevent further regression (Table 14-2).

Figure 14-13 accurately illustrates the suggested FML treatment cycle for overcorrection.

Management of Overcorrection—Case Example

The patient was found to be overcorrected by more than the desired amount at the 10-day postoperative evaluation. The steroid drops were tapered from five times per day to two times per day for 1 week and one time per day for 1 week. At the 2-month evaluation the refraction was close to plano and the steroid drops were restarted at three times per day for 1 month, two times per day for 1 month, and one time per day for 1 month.

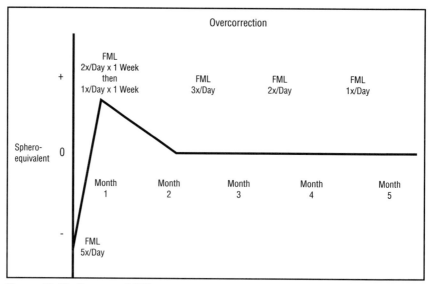

Figure 14-13. Suggested FML treatment cycle for overcorrection.

Presbyopia

Clinical Features

If a patient is overcorrected, presbyopic symptoms may be produced following the procedure.

Management

Reading glasses may be required, even though the patient did not require correction to read prior to the procedure.

Regression With or Without Haze

Clinical Features

Regression is more likely to occur with higher degrees of myopic and/or astigmatic correction. Factors that may lead to regression include preoperative flat K's, small optical zones, single zone treatment, high myopia, and steep wound edges. Another factor that can lead to regression is secondary UV exposure. Anecdotal reports have indicated regression after intense UV exposure. UV-related regression is most likely to occur in the first 6 months with exposure to unfiltered sunlight at a high altitude such as when skiing.

Management

If regression occurs, steroid drops are either increased in frequency or

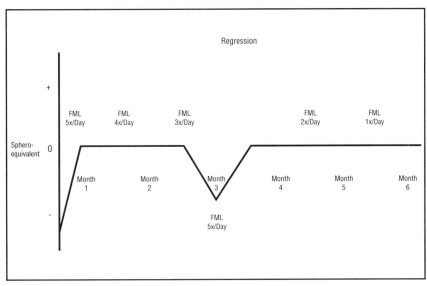

Figure 14-14. FML treatment cycle described in regression case example.

restarted. If after a few months there is an improvement in the refractive error, the steroids are tapered. If the eye remains undercorrected, retreatment can be performed after the steroids have been discontinued and after the refraction becomes stable. Typically, retreatment is not considered prior to 6 months following the PRK procedure. As a precaution, it is advised that patients use UV-protective sunglasses during the first 6 months when exposed to sunlight at a high altitude.

Regression without haze can be managed with a PRK enhancement that is similar in technique to a primary procedure. If there is regression with mild haze, a transepithelial approach followed by a PRK for the residual refractive error can be performed. If there is regression with severe haze, then a no-touch technique using a PTK mode should be done. Any residual refractive error can be managed in the future with a PRK enhancement for myopia, astigmatism, and/or hyperopia.

Management of Regression—Case Example

The patient was noted to have regressed at the 3-month postoperative evaluation. The steroid drops were increased in frequency from three times per day to five times per day for a 1-month trial. At the 4-month postoperative evaluation the refraction was close to plano and the steroid drops were tapered to two times per day for 1 month and then one time per day for 1 month.

Figure 14-14 depicts the FML treatment cycle in the above regression case example.

General Awareness

Pregnancy

If a patient becomes pregnant prior to having PRK or at any time during the first year following the procedure, the doctor must be made aware because pregnancy can affect the healing response. Also, some medications may pose a risk to an unborn or nursing child.

Eye Sensitivity

Some patients experience continuing tenderness when rubbing their eyes. This sensitivity can continue for some period of time. Additionally, patients may continue to experience sensitivity to light. Such sensitivities tend to diminish with time as the healing process evolves and use of the eyedrops is discontinued.

Adapted from Stein R. *Laser-PRK*. Toronto, Canada: Beacon Eye Institute:34-53.

Retreatment

Excimer laser enhancements are easily performed after a primary PRK if there is haze, central islands, undercorrection, overcorrection, or a decentered ablation after other surgical procedures including RK, cataract surgery, and PK. A thorough understanding of the preoperative assessments, techniques, and postoperative management are essential to achieve satisfactory visual outcomes.

Enhancements Post-PRK

Enhancements after a primary PRK can be divided into two categories:
1. Undercorrections and/or regression with a clear cornea
2. Undercorrections and/or regression with corneal haze

For those patients with clear corneas, it is preferable to wait a minimum of 6 months after surgery, especially if the refractive error is changing. If a patient is undercorrected at 1 month and the refraction is stable, the surgeon may consider an earlier enhancement. It is important that all drops be stopped for at least 1 month prior to enhancement because some patients regress as soon as drops are discontinued.

The general rule for all enhancement procedures is that the longer one waits, the more confident one can be that the cornea is stable.

Surgical Technique

Mechanical epithelial removal using a spatula, rotating brush, or alcohol technique is performed. It is important to note that some patients who were plano after a primary PRK procedure then regressed will often be hyperopic early post-enhancement. As the epithelial thickness changes, their hyperopia resolves, sometimes taking up to 4 months. This is a normal condition requiring no extra treatment.

However, patients who were undercorrected after their primary procedure with a relatively stable refractive error are close to plano soon after the enhancement and tend to remain stable.

Corneal Haze

It is best to wait at least 12 months to treat patients with corneal haze. It is a general rule that the longer one waits for the haze to resolve, the better the prognosis and the easier it is to treat. Again, patients should be off all drops with a stable refraction before retreating.

Haze in high myopes, and rarely in lower myopes, may take up to 2 years to resolve. If the patient insists on additional treatment, then the surgeon must proceed carefully. A transepithelial or no-touch technique is preferred. In these eyes, the epithelium is often mixed with newly formed collagen, and, if all the epithelium is removed mechanically, the result is an irregular surface. It is best to use the laser on the epithelium as a masking agent to achieve a smoother surface.

The key to the technique is to keep the microscope light as low as possible, especially near the end of the epithelium removal. When the laser ablates the epithelium, a reflected blue fluorescence is created. Usually, when the stroma is reached, the blue fluorescence changes to a black appearance.

Eyes with significant corneal haze and collagen mixed in with the epithelium show a speckled blue-black appearance when the stroma is reached. At this point, the surgeon should stop the ablation, and the eye should not be touched. The refractive ablation should be performed immediately. A PTK with a transition zone (eg, 0.35 mm) is then used to remove the corneal haze. Any residual refractive error can be treated in the future.

With this technique, reports indicate only a 20% recurrence of haze occurs with retreatment.

Decentered Ablations

The best approach to correcting decentered ablations is to prevent them.

When treating them, however, it is best to treat the residual myopia and to decenter the ablation in the opposite quadrant. This is more of an art than a science.

In the future, masking agents that ablate at the same rate as the corneal stroma may be used to smooth the corneal surface. By molding the collagen compound with a rigid gas-permeable lens, a smooth anterior surface is created. The laser can be used to ablate directly through the masking agent to produce a spherical central cornea.

Central Islands

A central area of steepening of the cornea as detected by corneal topography following PRK is the most common topographical abnormality. We usually wait 12 months if there is a persistent, symptomatic central island before we retreat with the excimer laser.

First, we look at the topography map and see exactly how wide and steep the island measures. After mechanical epithelial removal, an ablation zone of <3.0 mm is used to flatten the island using PRK.

Post-RK Enhancements

Treating post-RK patients remains somewhat controversial. Generally, we are uncomfortable performing a PRK over an RK for a number of reasons. Some patients after RK will complain not only of poor vision due to undercorrection, but also of fluctuating vision and problems seeing at night. PRK enhancements will not improve night vision problems, nor can they correct visual acuity fluctuations. Enhancements only correct residual myopia. The patient may blame the PRK surgeon for not correcting the pre-existing vision problems caused by the RK.

Patients who have had four-incision RK who are undercorrected often do well with PRK procedures. Patients with 12 or more RK incisions tend to do poorly with a high incidence of corneal haze. The etiology for this is not known and may be related to a dellen-like effect due to corneal contour.

We do not perform PRK enhancements for patients who have had more than eight-incision RK. If the patient had eight-incision RK and if the pre-RK refractive error was <–6.00 D, patients usually do well with a PRK enhancement. However, if the refractive error was >–6.00 D, there is a greater incidence of central corneal haze.

Most RK undercorrections are ≤–3 D. For these eyes, we prefer the laser/scrape approach in which the laser ablates most of the epithelium; then a spatula is used to remove the residual debris. This approach is preferred over mechanical epithelial debridement because it is often very difficult to remove epithelium adherent to RK incisions.

Research indicates a fairly significant hyperopic drift in RK patients long term. Therefore, performing a PRK enhancement on an RK patient who is −1 D may not be in the patient's best interest.

Penetrating Keratoplasty

Eyes that have had a PK have a higher incidence (25%) of haze following PRK enhancements when compared with virgin corneas. These patients can do well, however, if they are myopes with regular astigmatism. If they have irregular or asymmetric astigmatism, then an AK is done to create more regular astigmatism, followed by PRK enhancement.

In the future, flying spot excimer laser technology, along with computerized videokeratoscopy, may be used to treat the steeper areas of the cornea to correct the irregular surface.

Post-Cataract Surgery

Excimer laser surgery can be used following cataract surgery, especially if an incorrect implant is used, thereby creating a significant myopic error.

One patient was referred to us 6 months post-cataract surgery with a −7 D refractive error due to an incorrect lens power, with a cataract developing in the fellow eye. We performed a PRK on the −7 D eye, resulting in a near plano refraction. Subsequently, the patient underwent successful cataract surgery in the fellow eye.

Complications

The main complication associated with enhancements is corneal haze, which occurs more commonly than in primary corneal procedures. Although decentered ablations are relatively uncommon, the incidence is also higher than in primary procedures, especially with mechanical epithelial removal techniques, because the patient's view of the red fixation light is often blurred. The surgeon must be aware of this and may need to hold the eye for proper fixation.

Retreatment Rates

We have had a 3.6% retreatment rate in our first 1000 eyes (36 eyes). Most were in the high myopia range and were undercorrected, underwent regression, and/or had significant haze. Excellent results were obtained with 85% of patients achieving an acuity of 20/40 or better uncorrected. Additional treatment can be performed if the patient is myopic and/or has recurrent haze.

Adapted from Stein R. Ophthalmologists need to understand preoperative assessments, techniques, and postoperative management to achieve satisfactory visual outcomes. *OSN*. 1996;Sept 15:38.

Other
Options

Chapter 16

Comparison of Radial Keratotomy and Photorefractive Keratectomy

PRK is the most recent entry into the field of refractive surgery. RK has been in use in the United States since the 1970s. In the RK procedure, diamond-tipped surgical knives are used to make a series of radial incisions into the cornea. The central surface of the cornea flattens out, resulting in the correction of myopia.

Surgical Technique

RK

The RK procedure to correct myopia was developed by a Russian ophthalmologist, Dr. Svyatoslav N. Fyodorov, at the Moscow Institute of Clinical Eye Surgery in 1973. He noted that a pilot who had injured his cornea with glass was found to have a marked reduction in his shortsightedness. Dr. Fyodorov, by performing thousands of RK operations, established a high rate of success. Later, hyperopia and astigmatism treatments were developed. Currently, thousands of RK operations have been performed in North America over the past 20 years by eye surgeons on millions of people throughout the world.

RK for myopia and AK for astigmatism are surgical procedures that use relaxing incisions to alter corneal curvature. This has been pioneered and popularized by Leo Bores, Spencer Thornton, and J. Charles Casebeer. Radial incisions cause a weakening of the peripheral cornea, which permits the normal IOP of the eye to push the peripheral cornea outward, causing the central cornea to flatten (Figure 16-1).

A number of factors influence the results of RK. The first is the diameter

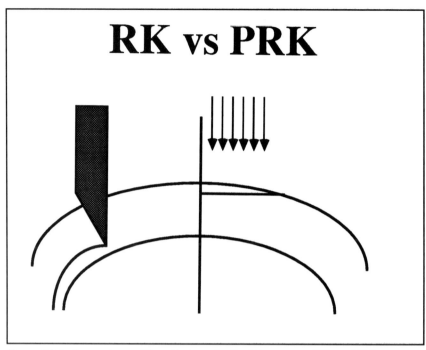

Figure 16-1. Comparison of the effect on depth of the cornea (RK vs. PRK).

of the central clear zone, which is usually between 3.0 and 4.0 mm. Smaller diameter clear zones produce greater flattening of the cornea than larger zones, but smaller zones may produce glare at night when the pupil dilates. The younger the patient, the larger pupil can become a problem.

The second variable is the number of incisions, which usually varies from four to eight, four giving approximately 75% of the effect achieved with eight. Most of the flattening of the central cornea is achieved with four or eight incisions; succeeding incisions have progressively less effect.

The third variable is the depth of incisions; deeper incisions produce greater central flattening. A greater amount of myopia requires a smaller clear zone, deeper incisions, or more incisions. There is an upward limit of diopters of myopia that this procedure can affect.

Individual patient response to the incisions is an important factor to RK results. Considerable variables include:

- **Age**—older patients experience a greater correction
- **Sex**—females require more surgery
- **Corneal curvature**—the steeper the cornea, the greater effect
- **Corneal thickness**—if the cornea is thick there is a greater effect

Some of the instruments and techniques utilized differ from surgeon to surgeon. The style of diamond knife blade and configuration of the knife footplates, the accuracy of ultrasonic pachymeters, the control of fixation instruments, the direction of the incisions, and the manual technique of making each incision are all variables in RK that affect the results. There is also inherent biological variation in healing among individual patients.

Comparison of RK and PRK

- **Predictability**—RK has a long learning curve for the surgeon before one obtains the required predictability (Table 16-1). PRK, on the other hand, is computer driven, and not affected by as long a learning curve. Optimum predictability will be achieved as long as the appropriate safety checks are performed, data input to the computer are accurate, and the bed is adjusted accurately for centration of the procedure. With RK, knives may become degraded and chipped, causing a variability in the predictability. However, laser optics could also become dull and reduce the predictability.
- **Need for retreatment**—Undercorrection is common with RK. Retreatment ranges from 10% to 50%, depending on the surgeon, and many patients have multiple retreatments. The need for retreatment is much lower with PRK, ranging from 5% to 10% in patients with >6 D of preoperative myopia.
- **Surgical accuracy**—Surgeons performing PRK can rely on the accuracy of the computer, rather than a hand-held blade, which can vary with different surgeons and their techniques.
- **Degree of correction**—RK can succeed in cases requiring only up to 6 D to 7 D of correction. However, PRK can produce up to 15 D of correction comfortably. Larger corrections with PRK can lead to an increased incidence of haze.
- **Rehabilitation**—The results of RK are quicker; patients are rehabilitated almost the next day and can return quickly to work. Patients are almost immediately gratified, even though there may be a regression in the future that requires a secondary procedure. These patients return immediately to the workplace and soon stimulate interest in others to have the procedure (this is similar to Laser Assisted In Situ Keratomileusis [LASIK]). With PRK, visual recovery is usually within 4 to 5 days, but in some cases may take up to 2 to 3 months. Patients require psychological support, as they are often slow to recover their full spectacle-free vision.
- **Long-term results**—RK has a long track record, with long-term results known, while PRK does not yet have long-term results.

	PRK	RK
Table 16-1. **Comparison of PRK vs. RK**		
Technique	Laser energy	Diamond blade
Control	Computer	Hand-held
Depth	Superficial	Deep
Location	Central	Peripheral
Stability (low myopia)	Excellent	Good
Recovery	Slower	Quick
Structural Integrity	Excellent	Weakened
Fluctuating Vision	Minimal	Common
Experience	10+ years	20+ years

- **Cost**—In terms of financing, RK will always be less expensive, as there are minimum start-up costs. PRK involves the capital cost of the laser and, at present, high maintenance costs. Conversion to solid-state lasers would at least reduce maintenance costs.

Side Effects

- **Glare**—The side effect of glare around headlights is common to both procedures if pupillary size is not determined at the outset (Figure 16-2). Glare is relatively short-lived for both procedures. RK patients are aware of starbursts around lights and glare, which is worse when surgeons utilize an excessive number of incisions or an optical zone smaller than 3.0 mm. Some RK patients may experience glare for about 5 months, which then gradually decreases over time. Some PRK patients have glare because some degree of reticular haze involving the visual axis is present. This haze decreases with time for most patients but there can still be residual haze that reduces best-corrected vision and contrast sensitivity. A repeat laser procedure may be required to remove the haze.

- **Haze**—PRK affects the central portion of the cornea and can produce haze which may interfere with vision. RK leaves the center of the cornea untouched.

- **Astigmatism**—After RK, there is a significant increase in astigmatism in a small number of patients due to scar contracture, while after PRK only a slight increase in astigmatism occurs rarely.

- **Visual loss**—In RK, only the peripheral portion of the cornea is invaded by incisional cuts, with the central zone unaffected. Loss of vision is rare. In PRK, the central portion of the cornea is affected by treatment, so loss

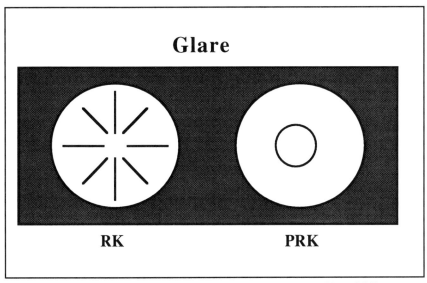

Figure 16-2. Glare can be produced with a small optical zone in RK or PRK.

of vision is a possibility, although it occurs only rarely.

- **Fluctuating vision**—In RK, the cornea is permanently weakened as the cuts have to be more than nine tenths the thickness of the cornea to achieve the flattening effect required, often resulting in a fluctuation of postoperative vision. Thirteen to 31% of RK patients undergo a progression of the refractive effect toward hyperopia that continues for years (Figure 16-3).
- **Pain**—PRK causes considerably more pain than RK. The use of nonsteroidal anti-inflammatory drugs and bandage contact lenses have significantly reduced the pain after PRK to the same level as RK.
- **Infection**—After RK, serious complications rarely have been reported, but there have been cases of endophthalmitis. In contrast, we have experienced no infections after PRK.
- **Perforation**—With RK, there is always the danger of perforation, both micro and macro, increasing the danger of endophthalmitis. On the other hand, PRK does not enter the anterior chamber, and consequently intraocular inflammation and infection should not occur.
- **Structural integrity**—After RK, the cornea is structurally weakened. For this reason, cases of rupture of the cornea secondary to blunt trauma have been reported. On the other hand, PRK does not alter the cornea's structural integrity, so PRK will withstand greater external pressure in the event of an injury (Figure 16-4).

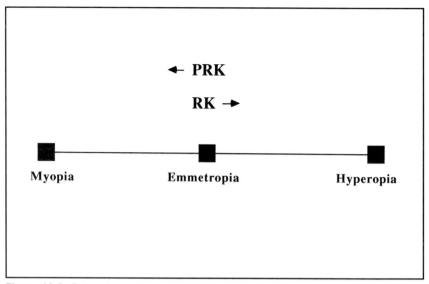

Figure 16-3. Refractive error can shift following refractive surgery. In PRK, the shift over a 6- to 12-month period is toward myopia for which additional treatment can be performed. In RK, the shift is toward hyperopia which can occur even years following surgery.

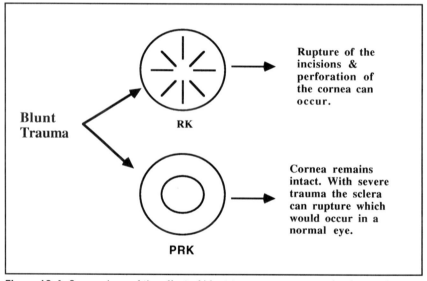

Figure 16-4. Comparison of the effect of blunt trauma on a cornea that has undergone RK and PRK.

Discussion

In comparing PRK with RK, it is our opinion that PRK is the winner. PRK is much more user-friendly for the surgeon and has a shorter learning curve.

For the patient, the word laser is is much more acceptable over a cutting procedure as it connotes high technology and safety. We feel that whenever the excimer laser is available, RK will gradually disappear in the community.

RK may still have a limited role in:

- Reoperation for enhancement in low (<2 D) residual myopia where one wants to obtain a dramatic, quick result with the mini-RK procedure.
- For repeat of an asymmetric cornea if one wants to do asymmetric RK surgery based on corneal topography.

Laser Assisted In Situ Keratomileusis

LASIK is gaining increasing popularity for several reasons. The controversy of whether surface PRK or LASIK gives better results with less downside risk is being debated at present. Each has its advocates. Meanwhile, growing interest among ophthalmologists has given rise to many new microkeratomes from several companies. Some of these keratomes are manual (Moria, Guimarães); others are automated (Chiron Vision, Phoenix, SCMD). The classic keratome and role model is the Chiron microkeratome. Newer keratomes address safety in lifting the corneal flap.

While perhaps only 5% to 10% of ophthalmic surgeons will be doing LASIK because of the longer learner curve and the increased risks, no laser book is complete without some discussion of LASIK. However, this book is devoted primarily to surface PRK excimer laser and is not a detailed text on LASIK. There are many advantages of LASIK as mentioned in Table 17-1. The most convincing is the fact that there is minimal or no pain associated with LASIK. There is also rapid recovery so the patient is seeing well soon following surgery. In addition to that, they eye looks extremely normal the day following surgery. It is often most difficult to tell where the corneal flap has been laid down.

Historical

Dr. Jose Barraquer developed keratomileusis, which was a stepping stone to the current LASIK, in the late 1940s. While the technique of keratomileusis was ingenious in its concept, it did not produce the expected surgical and functional results. It was also mechanically very cumbersome.

Table 17-1.
Advantages of LASIK

- Rapid recovery of vision
- Absence of pain
- No removal of Bowman's layer or epithelium
- Stable vision
- Long-term steroids not required
- Haze rare

In 1987, Dr. Jorge Krumeich modified Barraquer's classic technique to a no-freeze refractive surgery procedure. This was a giant step forward. Dr. Luis Ruiz of Bogota, Colombia, took the concept one step further and produced a refractive cut in situ. Ruiz then introduced automation of the microkeratome which simplified the procedure enormously and eliminated some of the common complications. Standardization still had not arrived.

In 1988, Dr. Gholam Peyman patented the idea and concept of doing intrastromal ablation on the cornea using the excimer laser. In 1989, Dr. Ioannis Pallikaris and his colleagues of Crete, Greece, studied the effect of the excimer laser or rabbits' eyes after lifting a flap of anterior cornea. He used a corneal hinge of the lamellar flap. This hinge was a major contribution at the time. This reduced the risk of displacement of the lamellar flap, reduced the need for sutures, and avoided induced astigmatism. In 1989, he applied it to a blind eye and published a report in 1990. Dr. Lucio Buratto of Italy was the first to report a series of patients with successful LASIK results. In 1993, Dr. Guillimero Averos introduced a sutureless technique. This procedure was fast and less traumatic and facilitated anatomical healing and shortened recovery time. At this time, the technique of excimer laser ablation became more and more perfected so that multizone/multipass treatments and perfect centration became easier to accomplish. New keratomes, automated and manual, are being developed to meet the rising interest in LASIK. New changes are currently being made in which the flap is hinged superiorly instead of medially. This conforms with eyelid movements.

Surgical Technique

Preoperatively, proparacaine 0.5% is used to anesthetize the cornea along with an antiobiotic drop. A methylcellulose sponge soaked in proparacaine and held for 45 seconds in the fornix helps the anesthesia. Powderless gloves are used. Be sure the lashes and eyelid do not interfere with surgery. Insert lid speculum. Place alignment marks on the cornea with methylene blue.

The IOP is raised to 65 mmHg with a suction device that elevates the cornea. The microkeratome is applied usually to a 160 μm depth and a cornea flap is lifted by the smooth forward movement of the microkeratome. A small hinge is left at the medial aspect. The stroma is laid bare by reflecting the corneal flap. With careful centration, a central area of the stroma is ablated with the excimer laser to correct the myopia and astigmatism. In the case of hyperopia, a larger corneal flap is required. The stromal bed is cleaned and the corneal flap is replaced. It adheres within a few minutes to the underlying bed.

Advantages

For the patient the results are almost instant. There is rapid restoration of vision. Nomograms for the laser for accurate refractive error correction are now being developed for each of the different excimer lasers available. There is absence of pain as the epithelium is left intact. This results in great patient acceptance and word of mouth support for the procedure. There is minimal haze effect. Steroids are unnecessary in minimizing the concern of induced cataracts and secondary glaucoma. The postoperative course is short.

Disadvantages

Complications can occur. When they do occur, they can be much more serious than the complications of PRK. Perforation of the cornea with damage to the iris, lens, and ciliary body represents the most serious complication. There is a learning curve of 25 to 50 eyes for each surgeon in which there may be an increased number of complications and aborted surgery. Even when doing LASIK one should do a significant number each month to keep in practice. Even with experience, flap complications can occur. In high myopia, the depth of ablation when one starts at 160 or 130 μm may come close to creating ectasia or damaging endothelial cells. In order to limit the depth of ablation with higher degrees of myopia, smaller optical zones are chosen which can result in halos, especially at nighttime. In addition, the raising of the IOP to 65 mmHg, particularly in a high myope, may cause retinal hemorrhages or vein thromboses in an already

---

Table 17-2.
Problems with LASIK

- Misalignment of corneal flap
- Irregular astigmatism
- Interface problems between graft and host (debris, vessels, epithelial cells)
- Under- or overcorrections due to algorithm inaccuracy of excimer laser
- Induced astigmatism
- Halo vision, starbursts
- Night vision disturbance
- Retinal hemorrhage
- Need to abort if malfunction of keratome
- Surgeon dependent

---

compromised retina. This is even more likely in beginners when the pressure is sustained over a longer time.

However, LASIK does have its own subset of complications (Table 17-2). The patient repeat rate is still high (20% to 40%) and in addition to that the predictability is still not quite as accurate due to the fact that all the algorithms have not been well worked out for individual excimer lasers. There also may be mechanical problems that occur at the time of surgery. These include those noted in Table 17-3. Of the most disastrous are that there may be a loss of the footplate and complete uncapping of the corneal dome and cutting of the crystalline lens by the heavy suction that is being applied. Retinal hemorrhages may occur with 65 mmHg required and released on an already compromised cornea in higher myopes.

Selection of Patients

Many LASIK surgeons have used LASIK for -6.00 D to -25.00 D. Others have lowered the dioptric power to -1.00 D. Some reserved the procedure for myopia >10.00 D. Others avoid LASIK in >15 D myopia.

Technical Aspect of LASIK

LASIK is a technical advance over automated lamellar keratoplasty (ALK). An automated (or manual) microkeratome is used to create an initial corneal cap. This is usually hinged at the nasal aspect. Unlike ALK in which there is a second pass with a microkeratome, an excimer laser is used to ablate a specified amount of corneal stroma. The laser is used at 160 μm deep in stroma and provides a precise way to ablate the stromal layers.

The technique is ever-changing as new microkeratomes are being

---
Table 17-3.
LASIK Mishaps

- Loss of suction
- Microkeratome malfunction
- Improper seating of the flap
- Retinal hemorrhages from suction
- Loss of the footplate with disastrous complications
- Thick-thin areas of cap
- Corneal interface problems with epithelial debris

---

developed. Today the most popular model is the Chiron Automated Lamellar Microkeratome. In development states are the Phoenix microkeratome, the Schwind microkeratome, the Brazilian microkeratome, and the microkeratome of Moria Company of France.

Of importance after lifting the hinged corneal flap and applying the excimer laser centrally is to replace the flap in exactly the same place. Guiding markers on the corneal flap are important. After a period of 2 to 3 minutes, the corneal flap adheres permanently to its bed. It is important that the flap adhere well in its complete circumference. Why it sticks has been postulated to be due to surface tension and the inherent stickiness of the collagen growth substance of the cornea. When seen the next day, visual improvement is immediate and pain is non-existent or minimal (Figures 17-1 and 17-2).

Follow-Up

Prudent follow-up shortly after the procedure is required to be sure the cap does not get displaced. Follow-up the first few days may be important to recognize early complications. LASIK postoperative includes antibiotic for 1 week, steroid four times a day for 1 week, and artificial tears several times daily. Patients should be seen the day following surgery, at 3 weeks, and at 1, 2, 3, and 12 months later.

Discussion

There may be serious and severe complications in the first 25 eyes in the learning curve. Most experienced LASIK surgeons admit to a serious complication of one in 700 patients.

LASIK is technically more complex. The trade-off for a clear cornea, absent pain, and rapid recovery of vision with LASIK is the increased risk of a potentially more serious complication than can occur with PRK. Many have reserved LASIK for >8 D of myopia and PRK for <8 D but

Figure 17-1. The corneal flap is elevated with a microkeratome (top). Excimer laser ablates the central stroma to a prescribed depth (center). The corneal flap is restored (bottom).

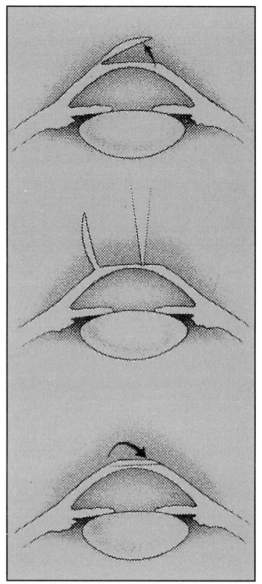

undoubtedly many will lower the indications to lower degrees of myopia for LASIK.

Will LASIK Replace PRK?

At the time of this writing, LASIK is generally being used primarily for the higher degrees of myopia and PRK technique employed for lower degrees. For some LASIK surgeons, LASIK is applied to all levels of myopia. The results in successful cases are dramatic for many patients. Providing a mixed message and discussing both LASIK and PRK to the same patient is often cumbersome and frequently ends in the patient not

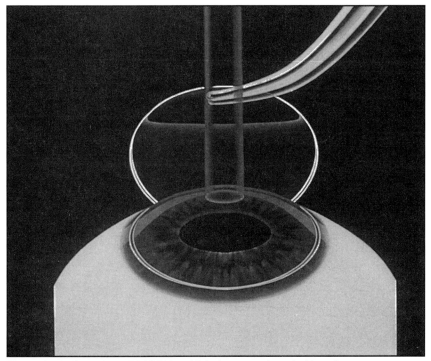

Figure 17-2. Side view of LASIK in which the corneal cap is hinged.

making a decision but wanting to wait. The question of the patient is often
"What would you do, Doctor?" when a mixed message is presented. Major
complications of eccentric ablations, flap irregularities, cutting errors, and
epithelial ingrowth occur at all levels, but the complication rate is minimal
with PRK for errors <7 D. As new microkeratomes are developed, there
may be a great future for LASIK in the hands of ophthalmic surgeons and it
may gain superiority in refractive surgery of all errors. Theo Seiler, the
American Academy of Ophthalmology 1996 Barraquer lecturer, stated that
he cannot justify LASIK for lower levels of myopia and higher levels to an
upper limit of 12 D because one should retain an unablated base of 200 μm
to prevent corneal ectasia.

Chapter 18

Other Options for Refractive Surgery

efractive errors such as myopia, astigmatism, and hyperopia can be treated by non-surgical procedures as well as refractive surgery, which includes any operation intended to alter the refractive state of the eye.

Correction for Myopia

Non-Surgical Procedures

For centuries voodoo, herbal medicine, and other superstitions were used to try to improve sight prior to the introduction of spectacles. When spectacles were introduced by Salvatore d'Avant in the 13th century, he was damned as the designer of the devil. He probably replaced an industry of myopic scribes at that time. On his tombstone is written "Here lies Salvatore d'Avant, the inventor of spectacles. May God forgive his sins." Spectacles did not gain wide acceptance until the 17th century. Non-surgical procedures include spectacles, contact lenses, orthokeratology, and cycloplegic agents.

Orthokeratology

Orthokeratology was developed in the early 1960s by optometrists in clinical practice. This procedure involves the use of specially designed rigid contact lenses which gradually reshape the front surface of the cornea. The lenses are somewhat flattened, and as the cornea adapts to the fit of the contacts, its curvature is flattened, reducing myopia and improving uncorrected visual acuity. Other lenses with gradually decreasing curvatures are then fitted, until the cornea has reached its optimum curvature.

Table 18-1.
History of Refractive Surgery

Year	Author	Surgery
1890	Fukala	Removal of the lens for high myopia
1894	Bates	Keratotomy for astigmatism
1898	Lans	Keratotomy for astigmatism
1949	Barraquer	Keratophakia and keratomileusis
1953	Sato et al	Anterior and posterior keratotomy
1972	Fyodorov and Durnev	Anterior RK
1979	Werblin and Klyce	Epikeratoplasty
1983	Trokel et al	Excimer laser
1987	Ruiz	Automated keratome developed
1988/89	Peyman and Pallikaris	LASIK

At the end of the treatment, "retainer" lenses are often prescribed to stabilize the improvements, even if the myopia has completely disappeared.

Refractive Surgeries

The ideal refractive surgical procedure should provide predictable, adjustable, and stable correction without any loss of corrected visual acuity.

Refractive surgery was first proposed a century ago (Table 18-1). There are many procedures to treat myopia (Table 18-2). This great number of surgical procedures reflect that so far none is the ideal refractive surgery.

Refractive procedures include keratoplasties, such as keratomileusis, epikeratoplasty, lamellar keratoplasty, ALK, RK, AK, PRK, LASIK, intracorneal lenses, clear lens extraction, and lens implants in phakic eyes (see Tables 18-1 and 18-2).

Epikeratoplasty

Developed by Werblin and Kaufman in 1981, epikeratoplasty for myopia involves the removal of a lamellar disc from a donor cornea, carving it on a cryolathe or die to form the concave lenticule, placing it on the surface of de-epithelialized recipient cornea, and suturing it into a peripheral circumferential groove or incision. This procedure flattens the central corneal curvature and decreases refractive power (Figure 18-1).

The predictability, like keratomileusis, is poor, and about 30% of patients lose some best-corrected visual acuity. Over- and undercorrection are frequent; only 59% achieve a refractive error within 3 D of emmetropia.

Table 18-2.
Surgical Procedures to Treat Myopia

Refractive Keratoplasty

Lamellar Techniques
    Keratomileusis
    LASIK
    Epikeratoplasty
    Intracorneal lens
    ICR
    Lamellar keratoplasty

Refractive Keratotomy
    RK
    Transverse keratotomy for astigmatism

Excimer Laser (PRK)
PK
Intraocular Implants
    Aphakic IOL, after lensectomy
    Phakic IOL

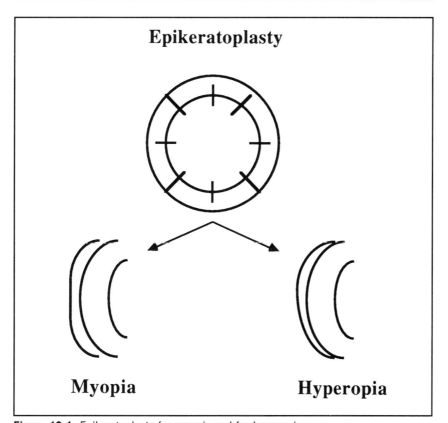

Figure 18-1. Epikeratoplasty for myopia and for hyperopia.

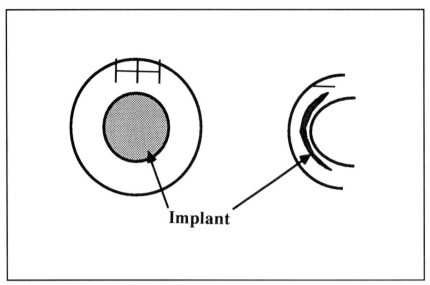

Figure 18-2. Intracorneal lens—Polysulfone.

The lenticule may be removed. The reversibility of the surgery is an advantage. The complications are irregularities of the corneal surface, loss of transparency, irregular astigmatism, epithelial ingrowth, and secondary microbial infection.

Intracorneal Lenses

There are two types of synthetic materials of intracorneal lenses: lenses with high refractive index materials—the polysulfone, and lenses from hydrogel. Both techniques were developed in 1981 and are still in the investigational stages.

Polysulfone is a material that has a refractive index of 1.633. This technique does not involve opening the eye, nor does it involve the use of the microkeratome. The lenticule can be implanted by placing it in a corneal pocket (Figure 18-2). The most important complication is aseptic necrosis of the cornea.

For hydrogel intracorneal lens implantation, it is necessary to remove a corneal disc with the microkeratome, place the lens on the corneal bed, the disc of cornea back into position, and suture (Figure 18-3). The hydrogel's lenticule changes the cornea's radius of curvature. Because hydrogel has a high water content, and thus is permeable to water and nutrients, it is a more successful material for intracorneal lenses.

Intrastromal Corneal Ring

The intrastromal corneal ring (ICR), developed in 1978 by KeraVision of Santa Clara, California, and Dr. David Schanzlin, is an optically clear ring

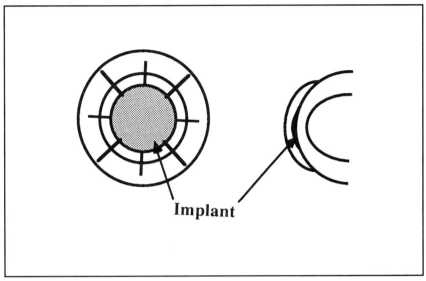

Figure 18-3. Intracorneal lens—Hydrogel.

approximately 6 to 7 mm in diameter. The ring is designed to fit into a circumferential intrastromal pocket that is surgically created in the peripheral cornea (Figure 18-4), creating an increase in the volume of the peripheral cornea and flattening the curvature of the central cornea. The major advantage is that it is a reversible procedure; it does not depend on wound healing for predictability, and it avoids the central cornea. It is useful for low degrees of myopia.

IOLs

There are two types of phakic lens implants:

1. IOLs that lie in the anterior chamber
2. IOLs that lie in the posterior chamber

Implanting an IOL in the anterior chamber of the phakic eye to correct myopia (Figure 18-5) was proposed by Strampelli in 1954. Joaquin Barraquer in Spain during the 1950s had experience with these implants, and abandoned the idea due to complications. George Baikoff and Albert Galant have resurrected this approach for the high myope, with lens designs of negative power.

The principal problem with this procedure is the trauma to the corneal endothelium resulting in corneal edema. Other complications are damage to the crystalline lens causing cataract and damage to the anterior chamber angle causing glaucoma. Recently modified lens designs may better preserve the endothelium and reduce complications.

Staar Surgical is investigating a posterior chamber phakic lens made of

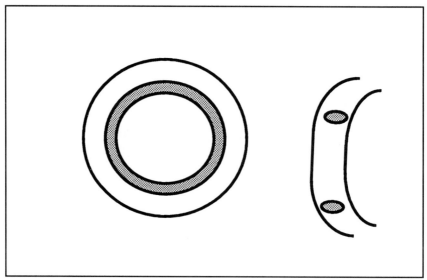

Figure 18-4. ICR.

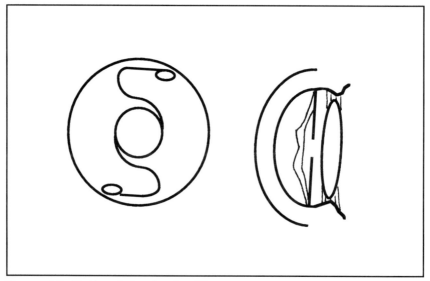

Figure 18-5. Phakic anterior chamber IOL.

collagen, from a design by Fyodorov. The lens, which the company is calling an implantable contact lens, is designed to rest on the surface of the capsular bag. A laser iridotomy must be performed preoperatively to prevent pupillary block glaucoma. Preliminary studies have been done in South America for high myopes, and results look promising.

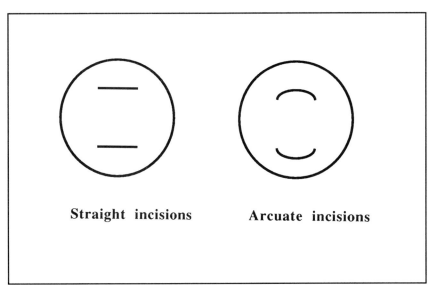

Figure 18-6. AK.

Astigmatism Correction

Transverse Keratotomy for Astigmatism

In transverse keratotomy for astigmatism, the cornea is partially incised with a diamond scalpel transversely on the steeper axis to flatten (Figure 18-6). The surgical procedure is usually performed under topical anesthesia, as in RK.

There are difference nomograms to treat astigmatism, changing the incision location, chord length, and degree of arc. Cuts can be straight or curved (arcuate incisions). Curved cuts are more predictable and create fewer problems with glare than straight cuts.

Hyperopia Correction

Hexagonal Keratotomy

There is currently no satisfactory procedure to correct hyperopia. HK, a procedure that places non-intersecting incisions in a hexagonal pattern around the cornea, offers one approach, but in one author's (HAS) hands and others there is a problem with predictability and induced irregular astigmatism. The procedure has been abandoned by the majority of surgeons.

Thermal Keratoplasty

The concept of TK dates back almost 100 years. Lans was the first to report that healing of the cornea could induce collagen shrinkage with resultant corneal curvature changes. In 1981, Neumann, Fyodorov, and Sanders described radial TK utilizing a nichrome wire that penetrates the cornea to 80% of its depth. The probe reaches high temperatures, producing necrotic corneal tissue at each burn site. The coagulations are radial, with eight rows of three or four applications each. At high temperatures, collagen and other molecules are thermally damaged and a healing response is induced, leading to collagen shrinkage.

If collagen shrinkage is performed in the periphery of the cornea, a flattening in the anterior cornea curvature will occur at the treatment site accompanied by a relative steepening in the central and paracentral cornea.

Because radial TK requires penetration of the cornea to 80% depth with a probe heated to 600° C, this technique has had difficulty controlling the coagulation profile and depth. For this reason, there was significant regression and lack of predictability.

Laser Thermal Keratoplasty

The holmium:YAG laser emits electromagnetic radiation in the infrared range at a wavelength of 2.1 μm. At this wavelength, the cornea exhibits efficient absorption capable of increasing the temperature of water, which in turn causes heat-induced shrinkage of collagen fibrils.

The holmium:YAG laser from Summit Technology operates with 300-microsecond pulses at a repetition rate of 15 Hz and a pulse power of approximately 19 mJ. Each treatment location receives 25 pulses, which raises the temperature of the collagen in that location to approximately 60° C. The Sunrise Laser Thermal Keratoplasty from Sunrise Technologies operates with chromium-sensitized thulium, and holmium doped yttrium aluminum garnet at 2.1 μm wavelength. Pulse energy varies from 100 to 300 mJ/pulse, with a repetition rate of five pulses per second.

The corneal collagen is treated with infrared laser energy and elevated to its phase transition temperature range, causing a change in the collagen from a triple helix conformation to a partly coiled state. This conformational change results in an immediate contraction of the fibers.

The laser energy delivery is accomplished through the objective lens of a specially modified slit lamp. The patient sits comfortably upright and is oriented by the standard head and chin rest of the slit lamp. The treatment pattern is centered on the patient's pupil, and consists of 16 spots (eight

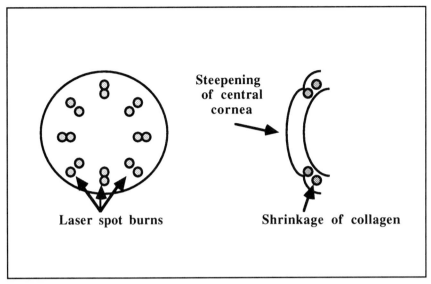

Figure 18-7. LTK.

rows with two radial spots each) with a variable diameter ablation zone
(Figure 18-7). The surgical technique is done under topical anesthesia.
Postoperative care involves topical antibiotics for 2 to 3 days.

A study by Seiler showed an average corneal steepening of 6.00 D was
achieved. The steepening effect underwent partial regression over the first 4
months and was felt to be stabilized around 6 months.

The advantages of holmium:YAG LTK include a consistent wedge-
shaped collagen shrinkage profile, no need to penetrate the cornea with a
heated wire, and a treatment temperature that shrinks collagen fibrils
without causing zones of tissue necrosis. Further follow-up is required to
determine stability of refraction.

Radio Surgery for Hyperopia

Recently, Mendez has developed a high frequency (300 to 500 MHz)
"radio" surgery for hyperopia. Working 7 mm from the optical center, he
claims the radio surgery provides better predictability for hyperopia than
LTK.

Summary

Many procedures are available to eliminate spectacles and contact lenses
to regain emmetropia for patients. We have reviewed the more popular
procedures. Our feeling is that the excimer laser, with or without lamellar
keratoplasty, will be the survivor.

Marketing Issues

Chapter 19

Marketing the Excimer Laser for Photorefractive Keratectomy

The battle for visual supremacy continues between proponents of RK, PRK, and LASIK. The target market is virtually the same: nearsighted men and women, ages 25 to 55, with annual household incomes of $30,000 or more. The only real difference is the method of surgical delivery.

The marketing strategies used to promote RK during the past few years have been highly successful in not only reaching this target market, but convincing patients to have the procedure done. Unfortunately, in some cases, they've been a little too convincing (ie, "Throw Away Your Glasses"), resulting in a recent flurry of negative exposure from the national media.

Reinventing the marketing wheel is not a prerequisite to an effective PRK campaign, which is true for even the inexperienced refractive practices that have never offered the benefits of refractive surgery to their patients. Thanks to extensive historical RK advertising campaigns on television and radio and in newspapers and magazines across the country, public awareness (and acceptance) of refractive surgery has never been higher. These campaigns have consistently proven that the public responds when presented with the right message, the right media mix, and the right price. They have also proven that refractive surgery is a market-driven product.

Even though similarities exist between RK, PRK, and LASIK marketing principles, practices must develop individual marketing strategies unique to their practice and demographic region. They must also develop a specific niche to help position themselves above their competitors.

Planning

Planning is important because of the ever-changing nature of marketing, especially in refractive surgery. It is important to plan for every phase of your campaign, before it becomes an issue. Your initial plan might focus on the fact that your practice is perhaps among the only group of ophthalmologists in your area who currently owns an excimer. What do you do when five or six excimers become available in your area? A strategy is needed.

What happens when your competitor drops his or her price to garner more market share, and you are finding it difficult to keep an adequate cash flow at $2000 an eye? How will your practice respond when a negative report by the media comes out regarding an overcorrected patient? What message will your campaign convey during this time period?

These are all scenarios that have to be addressed in your initial planning sessions. As we have witnessed in marketing refractive surgery during the past few years, advertising strategies shift quickly and are in a seemingly constant state of evolution. Your refractive marketing campaign will require constant attention and fine tuning. In putting together your initial marketing strategy, plan for change. Develop a flexible plan that allows you to change with the times. Be proactive, not reactive. When competition heats up, strengthen your position and give patients a reason for selecting your practice over your competitors. When prices start to drop (which they will), don't chase them down or you'll end up giving your services away. Promote the importance of quality care and the tremendous change the excimer is making in people's lives. Remind patients how priceless the gift of sight really is.

Other Concerns and Issues

In addition to planning, there are six other important areas to consider in putting together a successful marketing strategy for refractive surgery.
1. **Positioning**—Carve out a niche to influence public perception.
2. **Pricing**—Don't price yourself too far above or below the "market."
3. **Professional Relations**—Comanaging refractive surgery patients.
4. **Promise**—Don't make promises you can't keep. Be realistic. This invites disappointments and lawsuits.
5. **Proactive**—Be proactive in your marketing. Don't react.
6. **Philosophy**—Establish a marketing philosophy you're comfortable with.

Positioning

To separate your practice from its competitors, develop a marketing niche that positions you as a leader in the field. For instance, were you the first practice to purchase an excimer in your area? Were you the first practice to offer local patients the benefits of PRK? Does your surgeon have more recent training in PRK? Is your laser different or superior than others in your area? If you can't be first, then be among the first. If you can't be the most experienced, then be the most caring and professional. Somewhere in your practice lies a uniqueness that will enable you to strengthen your position in the market. If you are having difficulty finding your niche, your patients may be the answer. Ask them why they chose you for their eyecare and how satisfied they are with the care they received.

Pricing

PRK is a price-sensitive product. It has been proven time and again that patients respond to discounts and special pricing offers, especially when there is a substantial out-of-pocket expense involved. Unfortunately, campaigns based on price tend to have a downward spiraling effect which often results in prices you cannot afford to offer. Because of the high costs associated with operating the excimer (eg, gases, optics, maintenance, service fees), it is imperative that practices maintain their charges at profitable levels. Much of your pricing structure will be based on your position in the market. Mature practices with experienced refractive surgeons may have an easier time commanding higher fees than inexperienced refractive surgeons just starting out. To avoid price wars, focus your PRK campaign on benefits and advanced technology. As a reference, current prices for PRK are hovering at $2000 per eye and slightly higher for LASIK.

Professional Relations

Initial research and feedback from optometrists across the country indicate a much broader embrace of PRK in the optometric community than RK has enjoyed. If current levels of interest continue, optometrists will play a substantial role in the PRK market. Their involvement could range from simple patient referral to equity ownership in an excimer laser center. There is also an optometric movement underway to gain approval for allowing optometrists to perform PRK without the supervision or guidance of an ophthalmologist or any other medical doctor. Optometrists could become competitors or partners. Comanaging refractive patients with optometrists is working quite successfully around the country. They have been able to recognize complications and communicate with the original surgeon.

Unrealistic Promises

It is easy to create unrealistic expectations about PRK results. Many patients hear only what they want to hear. Any mention of 20/20 or perfect vision can lead the patient to expect that outcome. Although many patients may indeed enjoy 20/20 vision after refractive surgery, avoid making these promises. Instead use terms like "greatly improved vision" for the higher myopes, or "you could enjoy near perfect vision" for patients with mild to moderate myopia.

Prepare patients for dramatic results, and express these dramatic results during their early postoperative visits. When a patient who was 20/1000 comes in seeing 20/50 1 day postoperatively, that is a dramatic improvement. Show the patient the before and after difference on the eye chart, but do not show the 20/20 line. Inform the staff not to use phrases like, "You're only seeing 20/50, but that will probably improve in a few days, so I wouldn't be too worried at this stage." Instead, have them say, "Wow. Yesterday you were seeing 20/1000, and today you are already seeing 20/50." Such a statement does not mislead the patient, nor does it give false information. It is simply a more positive method to reinforce results.

Also, do not understate the possibility of a patient experiencing discomfort after the procedure. Many patients hear how painless the laser procedure is, and confuse that with the discomfort they will likely experience during the immediate postoperative period. It is better to overstate the possibility of postoperative pain, because the patient may actually experience very little discomfort.

Be Proactive in Your Marketing

Set your marketing sails on a course and stay as true to it as possible. It's okay to tack back and forth for better positioning, but avoid heading back into port at every sign of foul weather. Stick to the benefits of the procedure and the strengths of your practice. Prepare yourself for opportunities in the marketplace that allow you to shift focus without losing momentum. Be prepared for increased competition, pricing wars, and misleading campaigns, but don't focus on them.

Marketing Philosophy

Every practice has a level and style of marketing that its members are comfortable with. Some practices take the most aggressive, liberal strategy possible, while others appear more comfortable being passive and conservative. Whatever the case, don't develop a marketing philosophy you are not comfortable with. In all likelihood your marketing philosophy will change during the course of a campaign depending on results. The important thing to consider is an aggressive philosophy often results in more surgical volume in a shorter period of time. The conservative approach may win out in the long run, but you have to have the patience, time, and financial means to let the campaign run its course.

The High Cost of Miscommunication

After completing your marketing plan, attention should be directed internally to minimize potential miscommunication between staff members and patients. Misinformation can be one of the costliest errors your practice can make, and one of which you may never be made aware.

For example, in an effort to generate surgical volume for the excimer, a member of patient services slightly misstates the capabilities of the laser, and unknowingly creates an unrealistic expectation for a particular PRK patient. This staff member may also understate the risks involved with the procedure and the length and pain associated with postoperative recovery. When this patient comes in for an evaluation, a technician answers his or her questions in yet a slightly different manner. By the time the patient sees the doctor, the questions are answered in perhaps a more accurate light, which confuses the patient and leaves him or her uncertain of whom to believe.

At this stage, the patient's confidence in the procedure (and the surgeon) begins to wane, and a once favorable impression is quickly changed to one of uncertainty. More often than not, this type of miscommunication results in the patient avoiding confrontation by not expressing his or her concerns. The patient simply refuses to schedule and informs the doctors and staff he or she would like to think about the procedure a little more before having it done.

More often than not, this type of patient never schedules, which leaves the doctor wondering why such a good PRK candidate would choose not to have the procedure performed. Unless the doctor is made aware of the ongoing miscommunication, it is a difficult situation to rectify.

A worst-case scenario would be for the patient to actually schedule surgery and receive a nearly perfect result, but not as good as the staff in patient services promised. The patient might also experience a lengthier postoperative visual recovery and experience more discomfort after surgery than expected. This type of patient will never be completely satisfied, and in all likelihood will discourage others from having PRK. You may have increased your PRK volume by yet another patient, but in reality, you have probably cost the practice an additional five cases you would have received through normal referral patterns.

Avoiding Miscommunication Pitfalls

To avoid these types of miscommunication, establish an excimer laser or LASIK handbook for all staff members. Because no two practices are exactly alike, this handbook should not be generic. It should outline practice-specific information regarding the entire patient process for handling PRK patients. Included in this workbook would be the following:

- Triaging initial PRK patient inquiries—outlines what information should be communicated to the patient during the initial inquiry.
- The complete contents of your refractive "Patient Packet"—provides samples of the materials being sent to potential patients.
- Answers to commonly asked questions—provides staff with answers to questions regarding candidacy, risks, benefits, recovery, etc.
- Tracking and follow-up forms—informs staff what type of information will be needed each month for purposes of tracking and follow-up and shows a sample of each.
- Advertising samples—helps keep staff informed about what message is being conveyed by the practice to the general public.
- Informed consent forms—designed to educate staff members on the contents of the form and enable them to answer questions regarding it.

Introducing Refractive Surgery to Your Staff

Your staff needs to believe in the procedure and support your efforts wholeheartedly. Your staff may know what to say and do when it comes to performing surgery, but it is how they say and do it that really matters.

The best method for introducing your staff to PRK is to allow them to witness the tremendous change the excimer is making in people's lives. Have PRK patients discuss their life-changing stories at one of your staff meetings, and allow staff members to view the actual procedure and observe select postoperative examinations. If possible, have myopic staff undergo refractive surgery and become advocates.

Identifying Your Target Audience

The basic definition of target audience is the group of individuals who are most likely to respond to a particular product or service being offered.

The target audience for PRK or LASIK candidates is primarily the same audience that has been targeted for years for RK. The basic makeup of refractive candidates is:

- An almost even split between male and female
- Between the ages of 25 to 55
- Currently working outside the home
- Mild, moderate, or severe myopia
- Annual household income of $30,000 or more
- Tired of relying on glasses or contact lenses
- Contact lens intolerant
- Understands and responds to commercial messages
- Is busy and has little time to waste in a doctor's office with contact lenses
- Is inquisitive and consumer oriented
- Probably more litigious than cataract patients as refractive surgery is an elective procedure

Understanding Patient Psyche

Understanding a PRK patient's physical makeup and mental psyche helps to narrow the focus of your marketing strategy. The more narrow your focus, the more effective your message will be. A narrow focus also allows you to spend your advertising dollars more wisely, resulting in lower costs and higher response.

It does not make sense to target media whose listeners, viewers, and readers fall outside of these basic parameters. For example, if the top radio station in your market caters to the 12- to 25-year-old age group, it is not an ideal station for your message. Similarly, just because you get better rates for television during the day than during prime time, that doesn't make it a "good buy." The majority of PRK candidates work and thus do not view television from 9 am to 5 pm.

PRK patient characteristics cannot only help you plan your media buy, but also help you to treat these patients appropriately when they visit your office. Be appreciative of their busy schedule, and don't keep them waiting for hours for an initial PRK evaluation. Also, be aware of the growing litigious nature of today's patients, being careful not to create unrealistic expectations.

Advertising

Analysis

Before getting into excimer laser marketing, one has to analyze the nature of one's practice. Is it primarily a refractive or optometric type of practice? Is it primarily surgical? Is there a large contact lens component or is it a tertiary care practice comprised mainly of referrals? If there is a large refractive aspect and contact lens aspect to the practice, then one is in a much better position to get excimer laser or refractive patients from your practice. If you have a high surgical practice and low refractive practice, then in order to attract refractive patients one has to depend more and more on advertising and marketing.

It is imperative that your advertising message to the general public be accurate, ethical, and interesting. As important as accuracy and ethical content are to your advertising message, it must be interesting to grab the public's attention. Regardless of its accuracy, if your message fails to create a desire for the product and cause the public to take action, your campaign is destined for failure. Creating desire causes people to take action.

In promoting PRK, refer to PRK as the "laser alternative" to relying on glasses and contacts. Use phrases like "Reduce your dependence on glasses and contacts" or "Tired of relying on glasses and contacts?"

Refractive surgery has a high success rate, but very few people are able to "throw away" their glasses for the rest of their lives. Saying so would be a good example of creating unrealistic expectations. A practice should err on the conservative side, telling patients of the chance that glasses might be required after surgery for selective activities.

The Next Step in the Evolution of Refractive Surgery

Whether your practice has been performing RK for years or has yet to offer refractive surgery, the ideal way to market PRK or LASIK is to position the excimer laser as the next logical step in the evolution of refractive surgery. By mentioning that more than 1 million nearsighted men and women now enjoy freedom from their glasses thanks to refractive surgery, you create a proven base from which to launch the next phase in refractive surgery—the excimer laser.

Thanks to the success of laser procedures outside the realm of ophthalmology, the term laser has an extremely positive appeal to the general public. The more you use laser in your advertising, the more interest you will generate. Other phrases you might consider are "Computer-controlled for unparalleled accuracy" or "The most technologically advanced method for sight correction available today."

Implementing Your Plan

Implementing a marketing plan requires much more than calling up the media and placing a buy. Tracking systems should be in place well before the first print ad runs or the first radio commercial is aired. Follow-up systems should be in place to allow you to systematically keep in touch with patients between the time of their initial inquiry through the postoperative recovery period, as well as for those patients who never schedule. You want to know how many patients responded to each campaign, how many complete exams were scheduled, how many PRKs were performed, and exactly where in your system is everyone else who did not take action during this particular campaign.

If you're concerned your practice is ill-prepared to handle external promotions at this time, continue to prepare internally and save your advertising dollars for a later date. Otherwise, you are likely to overload your staff, upset new patients, and make mistakes you would normally not make under normal circumstances. Have role playing sessions and have the staff take turns playing the inquisitive patient. Go through every step of the process, especially with the telemarketing/patient service department.

Internal Marketing

The easiest type of marketing is in-house marketing where one looks at your own waiting rooms and your own office practice. Having the right combination of internal and external signs is very important. There should be illustrative pamphlets and brochures giving information about the refractive procedure that the patients can pick up in the waiting room area while waiting. A video is very important as a picture is worth a thousand words. The physician can target prospective cases by regular mailings. The most important philosophy is to plant many seeds and hope that in the future they will germinate.

It has been our experience that there can be intervals of 2 to 4 years from the time the seed is planted until it germinates and the patient returns for refractive surgery. Seminars can be very helpful in giving patients information about the different refractive techniques by having present three or four patients who have had the procedure done who can answer questions from the audience. It also gives prospective patients an opportunity to verbalize their anxieties and these questions can be answered by knowledgeable staff or patients who have had the procedure done. An informed and enthusiastic staff can make a big difference between success and failure as they can answer many questions that the patients have.

External Marketing

After internal marketing has been properly organized, one can then look at external marketing which involves print ads and the broadcast media where radio and TV spot ads may be used. As well, external mailings can go out to prospective patients. One can have a practice newsletter which is available at the office and which is distributed to new patients. A card identification program is very helpful. One can have name recognition or a corporate name or logo. This differentiates your practice from other practices. One can go to display cards and outdoor advertising on billboards. Community screening programs for example in malls and other public places can certainly introduce the subject of refractive surgery

Networking

Establishing a proper networking arrangement is very important between other ophthalmologists locally or within the state. Optometric referrals are very important as optometrists see the types of patients who can benefit from refractive procedures and they can refer these patients. They can be trained in proper pre- and postoperative follow-up and this varies from state to state as optometrists legally may perform different functions depending on the state. But, having a large optometric referral base can be very helpful in building up a refractive practice.

There may be other networking which can occur with other business groups or business agents or even large optical chains.

Financial Considerations

The financial considerations of getting into refractive surgery are very important and must be looked at very carefully. For example, the cost of a VisX laser with the astigmatism module was in the order of $500,000. One has to look at the cost of financing, the maintenance, which can be $40,000 per annum plus optics, which can range anywhere up to $40,000 per annum. The cost of a dedicated technician must be calculated into the equation as well as gases, royalty, or pillar point cards costs which may cost $250 per eye. There are many other miscellaneous costs that one must consider (eg, pharmaceuticals, bandage lenses, and other instruments).

One must have added staff retraining in order to keep the physician's staff up to date on queries on the excimer laser. Telephone skills must be refined to a very high level and the telephones must be answered promptly and efficiently or the benefits of the advertising will be lost. Interested patients must be scheduled to come in quickly to either see the physician or to see a trained technician. Other factors must be considered such as rent, insurance, malpractice insurance, depreciation of the laser, and new generation lasers.

Facts and Myths

There are many facts and myths with regard to refractive surgery and especially excimer laser surgery. First of all, in the United States the target market is 70 million myopes and maybe 40 to 50 million hyperopes. If 90% of the myopes have <6 D of myopia and each patient were to have 1.8 procedures (not everybody will elect to have both eyes done), and if 1% underwent PRK, there would be close to 1 million PRK procedures in the United States at $1500 to $2000 per eye. One can quickly see the megamillion dollar potential and the emergence of a new growth industry.

There are also many myths:

- That patients will line up at your door
- That this will be an answer to reduced Medicare payments
- That PRK is complication free
- That PRK is a guaranteed money maker

These myths are the furthest statements from the truth. If it is not run in a business-like fashion, PRK will be a guaranteed money loser and there will be many bankruptcies that will result.

Financial Conundrums

There are other financial conundrums in that one needs 25 to 30 cases a month to break even. With increased PRK volume there will be increased maintenance and optics costs. There will be increased gas and royalty costs, as well as increased advertising costs and increased staff.

Excimer Laser Participation

There are many arrangements whereby one can participate in an excimer laser. First, there are physician-owned excimer lasers, which are the ultimate where there are many participants and where there is a high volume of patients so that the costs of running the center can be minimal. In this way, the physician controls exactly what happens to the laser center and can make his or her own decisions.

Second, there are business-owned excimer lasers in which the corporate sector builds and provides the centers. There is a facility fee and a surgeon's fee. The excimer laser center is set up at a neutral and independent site. This has many advantages in that it allows new surgeons to participate in this exciting new technology without going through the costs of setting up an excimer laser facility and it enables many ophthalmologists and optometrists to participate in this exciting new technology. There are certain shortcomings in that it is business driven and there may be conflicts between what the business group wants to do and what the ophthalmologists and optometrists want to do.

Third, there are hospital-owned excimer lasers. In our experience, this has proven to be a disaster. Hospitals are not user-friendly. They have a lot of red tape. They do not provide evening or weekend service. Their budget for promotion competes with other departments. In our experience, hospital-owned excimer lasers have failed financially.

These are some of the considerations that every ophthalmologist must consider in depth before deciding whether or not to get involved in excimer laser surgery.

Future Trends

Improving Refractive Laser Therapy

The excimer laser represents the development of an exceptional technology. Ablation of the cornea with a change in the refractive error can significantly improve the lives of people wearing spectacles or contact lenses.

As experience with excimer laser photoablation progressed, surgeons began to recognize that some modifications were necessary. Surgical parameters such as increased diameter of the ablation, changes in the direction that the iris diaphragm opens or closes during the ablation, epithelial removal technique, multipass and multizone techniques, and eye fixation are constantly being modified.

The development of solid-state lasers may be the next advance to eliminate the expense and technical complexity required to operate the current machines that use expensive and toxic gases and complex optics to deliver the laser energy.

Excimer laser photoablation originally was expected to eliminate surgeon variability and create a minimal wound healing response on the part of the cornea. Because of surgical technique, laser factors, and/or wound healing, the outcome can be variable; one eye may have a perfect result and another eye with the same laser parameters may be under- or overcorrected. The laser beam homogeneity can vary from one laser manufacturer to another and also with the same make of lasers. In addition, laser factors (eg, fluence level, quality of optics) and surgical factors (eg, epithelial removal technique, degree of hydration) can vary, which may affect the outcome.

In reaction to the successes achieved worldwide with the PRK of myopia, studies of new techniques for correcting high myopia, irregular and asymmetric astigmatism, hyperopia, presbyopia, and other different applications of excimer laser surgery in ophthalmology are being done.

Corneal Trephination with the Excimer Laser

Laser trephination should theoretically improve the trephination precision and decrease post-keratoplasty astigmatism. The problem at present is the cost of this technology. Experimental corneal trephination has been achieved with the 193-nm ArF excimer laser. Compared with metal blades and other lasers, the 193-nm creates the best quality of corneal excision.

Of all laser and mechanical systems evaluated, the 193-nm excimer laser creates the most precise and regular trephined edges, the thinnest incisions, the least distortion of corneal tissue, and the least endothelial cell damage.

Optical delivery systems using an axicon lens, a rotating slit, and a computer-controlled scanning optical system have been developed for PK. With circular penetrating corneal trephinations and corneal grafts with the excimer laser, the corneas showed sharp, unbeveled cut margins with nearly perfect apposition of the inner wound aspects.

Asymmetric and Irregular Astigmatism

In the future, an ideal masking agent will be developed that could be used as an adjunct in excimer laser surgery for the treatment of asymmetric and irregular astigmatism. This agent would produce a smooth anterior surface prior to the laser procedure and ablate at the same rate as the corneal stroma. Probably a collagen compound will be the agent of choice.

It may be possible to apply this agent to the cornea and then mold it with a rigid contact lens of a known base curve. The laser could then be used to ablate through the masking agent to vaporize the cornea using a phototherapeutic mode. When the ablation has been completed through all areas of the masking agent, the laser procedure would be stopped. Theoretically, the post-laser corneal surface should have a similar curvature to the base curve of the contact lens.

The use of flying spot technology that is guided by computerized videokeratography has the potential to perform a custom corneal ablation to create a smooth spherical surface.

Presbyopia-Multifocal Ablations

The loss of accommodation with presbyopia or aphakia requires the use of multifocal lenses (spectacles, contacts, and IOLs) for the patient to see well at both distance and near. With the advance of excimer laser surgery, studies have been done to create a multifocal refractive effect of the cornea with excimer laser PRK.

To perform a multifocal ablation, a number of approaches have been used:

- Two concentric ablations, one at 6 mm and a second at 3 mm.
- Two ablations of 6 and 3 mm, with the smaller ablation decentered inferiorly by 2 mm.
- One single ablation in which the computer-controlled iris diaphragm is initially fully open to 6 mm and progressively closes until two thirds of the pulses have been delivered, leaving the periphery of the ablation zone flattened, but the central area measuring 3 mm in diameter, which has been blocked by a shield, with no intended refractive change. The ablations have been done on PMMA blocks and in rabbit corneas.

After multifocal ablations, a greater spread of surface powers is observed, often with a bimodal distribution, indicative of an apparent multifocal effect. More clinical studies are necessary to determine the quality of vision and the risks with this type of treatment.

As in the case of multifocal contact lenses or IOLs, quality of vision for both distance and near will be somewhat compromised. If patients are accepting of a reduced quality of vision in favor of requiring no optical aids, this approach with the excimer laser remains a possible useful modality in the future.

LASIK

LASIK is gaining popularity among eyecare professionals and patients. This initial wave of enthusiasm is common with the introduction of new surgical modalities. Future studies will be required to determine if this enthusiasm is justified based on objective data.

Potential advantages of LASIK over PRK include: less pain, rapid visual rehabilitation, early corneal stability, and less corneal haze. Because the epithelium is minimally disturbed, patients are generally comfortable in the early postoperative period. Visual acuity recovery is rapid since the epithelium is intact. Although regression can occur after LASIK, typically corneal stability is reached in 1 to 3 months. Because the epithelial-Bowman's complex is not affected, corneal haze is uncommon.

The potential advantages of LASIK have to be balanced with the potential risks. Complications of LASIK can vary from minimal to severe. The problems may be secondary to the microkeratome incision, the excimer laser, or the healing response. The most severe complication is intraocular penetration from the blade. This is an uncommon complication that may be seen if the footplate or depth-gauge is not set properly. The blade can penetrate the cornea, iris, ciliary body, or lens necessitating urgent surgical repair.

Other complications from the microkeratome incision include an incomplete flap or a free flap. Healing complications may include epithelial ingrowth, subluxated or dislocated flap, melted flap, or infection. Complications from the use of the excimer are similar to PRK with central islands, decentered ablation, or under- or overcorrection.

There are a number of concerns of LASIK that require further study. If a 160 μm flap is created, how much tissue can be safely removed with the excimer laser before creating ectasia? It is generally felt that a minimum of 200 μm of corneal tissue is to be left intact. Therefore, the maximum tissue ablated is 150 μm with an average corneal thickness. In order to treat high degrees of myopia (≥ 12 D), smaller optical zones must be chosen to decrease the depth of ablation. The problem with small optical zones (≤ 5 mm) is that there is a higher incidence of regression and halos, especially at nighttime.

The incidence of retreatments is higher with LASIK than PRK. The nomograms for LASIK are presently being developed. If, as has been proposed, the thickness of the flap can alter the refractive outcome, then the accuracy of the procedure with a single treatment will depend on consistency of flap creation.

The microkeratomes are undergoing refinements. There are many companies that have entered the market in selling different microkeratomes. The use of diamond or crystal blades may improve the accuracy. A shift from a gear system to propel the blade may allow easier cleaning. New proposed keratomes include a water jet or intrastromal laser to produce a cut.

Accuracy of refractive outcome and quality of vision are the most important long-term concerns. To date there are few studies that document 1-year LASIK results and complications. Quality of day and night vision should be subjectively and objectively assessed. The track record with PRK is more than 10 years. Controlled studies comparing LASIK and PRK using advanced excimer laser systems need to be performed. Information from these studies will allow eyecare professionals and patients to make informed decisions.

Discussion

It is clear that refractive surgery has reached the stature of the latest frontier in ophthalmology. Every indication suggests that by the year 2000 we will have a safe and predictable means of permanently correcting all types of refractive errors.

Future developments may result in lower costs for the surgeon and patient. Solid-state lasers may prove to have a lower operating cost by the elimination of toxic gases. Scanning and flying spot lasers permit a wider ablation and perhaps a reduced incidence of complications. The linking of computerized videokeratography with a flying spot excimer laser may allow us to create any corneal shape that we desire. The development of wound modulating drops to retain corneal clarity and prevent regression of effect will be an area of intense research in the years ahead.

Future considerations will delve into creating aspheric corneas from any regular or irregular cornea. In addition, alteration of the cornea may allow for the development of a bifocal surface.

The Future of Excimer Laser

- The development of LASIK to lift the epithelium and anterior stroma before using the excimer laser
- Eye tracking device to achieve more accurate centration
- Incorporation of data from computerized videokeratography into laser computer software
- Improved techniques for analyzing the laser beam to determine homogeneity
- Solid-state lasers to minimize gases
- Improved optics that are more resistant to degradation
- Larger optical zones
- Smoother transition zones
- Superior postoperative medication to modulate wound healing

Appendix I
Manufacturers

Aesculap-Meditec
23832 Via Monte
Coto De Caza, CA 92679
Voicemail/Fax: 714-589-6259

Aesculap-Meditec GmbH
Prussingstrasse 41
D-07739 Jena, Germany
49-364-16-53015, Fax: 49-364-16-53660

Autonomous Technologies Corp.
520 N. Semoran Blvd., Ste. 180
Orlando, FL 32807
407-282-1262, Fax: 407-282-9510

Chiron Vision Corp.
555 W. Arrow Hwy.
Claremont, CA 91711
909-624-2020, Fax: 909-399-1422

Coherent Medical
3270 W. Bayshore Rd.
P.O. Box 10122
Palo Alto, CA 94303-0810
415-858-2250, Fax: 415-857-0146

EyeSys Technologies, Inc.
2776 Bingle Rd.
Houston, TX 77055
713-465-1921, Fax: 713-465-2418

LaserSight Technologies Inc.
12249 Science Dr., Ste. 160
Orlando, FL 32826
407-382-2700, Fax: 407-382-2701

Nidek Co., Ltd.
6th Floor
Takahashi Bldg., No. 2, 3-chome
Kanda-Jinboucho
Chiuoda-ku
Tokyo 101, Japan

Nidek Inc.
47651 Westinghouse Dr.
Fremont, CA 94539
510-226-5700, Fax: 510-226-5750

Novatec Laser Systems Inc.
2237 Faraday Ave.
Carlsbad, CA 92008
760-438-6682, Fax: 760-438-7737

Summit Technology
21 Hickory Dr.
Waltham, MA 02154
617-890-1234, Fax: 617-890-0313

Sunrise Technologies
47257 Fremont Blvd.
Fremont, CA 94538
510-623-9001, Fax: 510-623-9008

VisX Inc.
3400 Central Expwy.
Santa Clara, CA 95051
408-733-2020, Fax: 408-773-7300

Appendix II

Guidelines for Patients Interested in Refractive Surgery

- Your suitability for refractive surgery will be determined by the ophthalmologist upon a complete evaluation. At this time all aspects of the surgery will be discussed and questions answered.
- A complete diagnostic work-up will be performed prior to surgery. This will include a computerized evaluation of the corneas (eg, a corneal topography).
- Patients wearing hard contact lenses should remove their lenses 3 weeks prior to the laser procedure.
- Patients wearing soft contact lenses should remove their lenses 72 hours prior to the laser procedure.
- The day of surgery you are required to come to the office 1 hour prior to the laser procedure for preliminary preparations.
- Patients must not wear make-up, particularly mascara and facial cream on the day of surgery.
- Before the procedure you will be provided with a discharge information sheet and should follow the discharge instructions as directed.
- During the PRK procedure, you will be able to wear your own clothes.
- You will not be given a general anesthetic, rather, the eye being treated will receive anesthetic eyedrops.
- Other eyedrops (eg, antibiotics and anti-inflammatory medicines) may be used as appropriate.
- Since allergic reactions are rare, please advise the ophthalmologist of any allergies you may have.
- You will be lying on your back during the PRK procedure.
- There should be little or no discomfort during the procedure. You will be able to ask questions and talk to the ophthalmologist during the process. Your surgeon will explain every step to you ahead of time.
- Your eyelids will be held open using an instrument called a speculum. This will prevent you from blinking.
- During the procedure, you will see a flash of light, hear a "ticking" sound, and notice distinctive smells.
- A bandage contact lens will be placed on the treated eye after the procedure. The top layer of cornea (the epithelium) heals during the first 2 to 4 days (it may take a little longer for farsighted people),

during which time vision will be very blurry and the eye will feel itchy. The eye may tear and be red and swollen. These are normal postoperative symptoms and will disappear within a few days. The contact lens will remain in place until the surface cells are healed. Keep in mind that younger people heal slightly faster. You are not permitted to drive during this period.

- The first 12 to 24 hours following surgery may be uncomfortable. The amount of discomfort experienced varies from patient to patient. The eye may be sensitive to light and sunglasses may be required.

- The institute will provide you with oral medication at the time of surgery in the event that you experience any discomfort or postoperative pain. You will have to purchase eyedrops for immediate and follow-up eyecare. A prescription can be given or a kit can be purchased from us for $30.

- Your vision will improve during the week following the surgery during which you will be able to return to your normal activities.

- You may experience difficulty with your depth perception at first while your eye heals. You may find that your focus will vary throughout the day and it may take a few seconds for objects to become clear. Your near vision will also be blurry until the eye heals. Age and severity of your refractive error will determine how long it will take your eyes to heal.

- We will need to see you postoperatively according to the following schedule:
One day after the surgery to monitor healing. Two or 3 days after surgery to remove the contact lens when the surface cells are healed. (This may vary from patient to patient depending on how the eye heals and may require further immediate follow-up.) The next follow-up visits will be specified by the doctor; usually it takes 2 weeks after the last visit and then once a month or every 6 weeks for 6 months.

Glossary

Absorption: Absorption is the process of atoms and molecules absorbing light. There are four interactions of laser light: transmission, scattering, reflection, and absorption. The most important interaction in excimer laser surgery is absorption of the laser energy by the cornea.

ALK: An acronym for Automated Lamellar Keratoplasty in which a microkeratome raises a corneal flap and then removes a portion of the stroma to reshape the cornea and correct refractive errors.

Atom: An atom is the smallest particle of a chemical element. They can exist alone or in combination with other atoms. In an atom the nucleus of protons and neutrons is surrounded by clouds of electrons with different energy levels, called electron orbitals.

Coherence: Coherence refers to light waves that are in phase. That is, their peaks and troughs are all coincident, thus reinforcing each other. A laser causes the light waves to be coherent, creating a much stronger beam.

Dimer: A dimer is a combination of two atoms. In the case of the excimer laser, the combination is a halogen (the fluoride gas) and an inert gas (the argon).

Electromagnetic spectrum: The electromagnetic spectrum is composed of a broad range of radiation, including ultraviolet radiation, visible light, and infrared radiation.

Excimer: The word excimer is a contraction of the words *excited* and *dimer*.

Fluence: Fluence or radiant exposure is a measure of the amount of energy flux per unit area at the surface of the material ablated, expressed as millijoules per square centimeter (mJ/cm^2).

Fluorescence: Fluorescence is spontaneous light emission by an excited atom.

Ground state: The ground state is the lowest energy state of an atom. An atom has an innumerable number of levels. If an atom is in the ground state and a radiation field containing photons of the appropriate wavelength is incident upon it, it can absorb a photon and go into the excited state.

Laser: An acronym of Light Amplification by Stimulated Emission of Radiation.

LASIK: An acronym for Laser Assisted In Situ Keratomileusis. A microkeratome raises a corneal flap and laser ablation is performed on the stroma and the corneal cap replaced.

Monochromaticity: Light of a single wavelength forms a specific color.

Monovision: Method of correcting presbyopia by having one eye corrected for near vision while the fellow eye is used for distance.

Photoablation: Photoablation or ablative photodecomposition means molecular break-up resulting from the absorption of high energy photons. The resultant molecular fragments are ejected from the surface at supersonic velocities. The excess energy is carried off, and there is minimal thermal damage in the residual tissue.

Photon: A photon is the smallest unit (quantum) of radiant energy.

Photoradiation: In photoradiation, light absorption results in a chemical change with alteration in molecular structure.

Photothermal interaction: In photothermal interaction, absorption of light results in increased molecular vibration and is converted to heat producing photocoagulation.

Pulse: A pulse is a brief change in electrical current or voltage.

Pulse duration: The duration of an excimer laser pulse depends on the short lifetime of the excited dimer molecule.

Spontaneous emission: When an atom is in an excited state, after some time the atom will spontaneously emit a photon of the same wavelength and return to the stable ground state (lower energy state).

Stimulated emission: When an excited atom is in an external radiation field of the appropriate wavelength, the atom can be induced or stimulated into emitting a photon and returning to ground state. The energy radiated by stimulated emission is in phase and coherent with the incident beam.

Wavelength: Wavelength is the distance in the line of advance of a wave from any one point to the next corresponding point. The wavelength of electromagnetic waves is the distance between successive peaks of the waves. In the case of the excimer laser, it produces radiation at the 193-nm wavelength in the "far-ultraviolet" portion of the electromagnetic spectrum.

Bibliography

Amano S, Shimizu K. Corneal endothelial changes after excimer laser photorefractive keratectomy. *Am J Ophthalmol.* 1993;116:692.

Ambrosio G, Cennamo G, De Marco R, et al. Visual function before and after photorefractive keratectomy for myopia. *Refract Corneal Surg.* 1994;10:129-136.

Anschutz T. *Ophthalmology Times.* April 1, 1994;19:7.

Arshinoff S, D'Addario D, Sadler C, et al. Use of topical nonsteroidal anti-inflammatory drugs in excimer laser photorefractive keratectomy. *J Cataract Refract Surg.* 1994;20(Suppl):213-223.

Assil KK, Quantock AJ. Wound healing in response to keratorefractive surgery. *Surv Ophthalmol.* 1993;38(3):289.

Barraquer JI. *Quertoplastie Arch Soc Am Oftal Optom.* 1961;3:147.

Bechara SJ, Thompson KP, Waring GO III. Surgical correction of nearsightedness. *BMJ.* 1992;305:813.

Bergman RH, Spigelman AV. The role of fibroblast inhibitors on corneal healing following photorefractive keratectomy with 193 nanometer excimer laser in rabbits. *Ophthalmic Surg.* 1994;25:170.

Binder PS. The excimer laser and radial keratotomy—two vastly different approaches for myopia correction. *Arch Ophthalmol.* 1990;108(11):1541.

Binder PS, Anderson JA, Rock ME, Vrabec MP. Human excimer laser keratectomy. Clinical and histopathologic correlations. *Ophthalmology.* 1994;101(6):979-989.

Bor ZS, Hopp B, Racz B, et al. Plume emission, shock wave and surface wave formation during excimer laser ablation of the cornea. *Refract Corneal Surg.* 1993;9(Suppl):S111.

Brancato R, Tavola A, Carones A, et al. Excimer laser photorefractive keratectomy for myopia: results in 1165 eyes. *Refract Corneal Surg.* 1993;9(Suppl):S96.

Brancato R, Tavola A, Carones A, et al. Excimer laser photorefractive keratectomy (PRK): first report from the Italian study group. *Ital J Ophthalmol.* 1991;3:189-195.

Buratto L, Ferrari M. Photorefractive keratectomy for myopia from 6.00 D to 10.00 D. *Refract Corneal Surg.* 1993;9(2suppl):S34.

Buratto L, Ferrari M, Rama P. Excimer laser intrastromal keratomileusis. *Am J Ophthalmol.* 1992;113(3):291.

Butuner Z, Elliott DB, Gimbel HV, Slimmon S. Visual function one year after excimer laser photorefractive keratectomy. *J Refract Corneal Surg.* 1994;10(6):625-630.

Campos M, Hertzog L, Wang XW, et al. Corneal surface after deepithelialization using a sharp and a dull instrument. *Ophthalmic Surg.* 1992;23(9):618.

Campos M, Nielsen S, Szerenyi K, et al. Clinical follow-up of phototherapeutic keratectomy for treatment of corneal opacities. *Am J Ophthalmol.* 1993;115:433.

Cantera E, Cantera I, Olivieri L. Corneal topographic analysis of photorefractive keratectomy in 175 myopic eyes. *Refract Corneal Surg.* 1993;9(Suppl):S19.

Carones F, Brancato R, Venturi E, Morico A. The corneal endothelium after myopic excimer laser photorefractive keratectomy [see comments]. *Arch Ophthalmol.* 1994;112(7):920-924.

Carones F, Brancato R, Venturi E, Scialdone A, Bertuzzi A, Tavola A. Efficacy of corticosteroids in reversing regression after myopic photorefractive keratectomy. *Refract Corneal Surg.* 1993;9(2 Suppl):S52-56.

Castanera J. Topographic comparison of monozone, multipass and multizone ablations for myopic photorefractive keratectomy. *Ophthalmic Surgery and Lasers.* 1996;27(5 Suppl):S471-S476.

Caubet E. Course of subepithelial corneal haze over 18 months after photorefractive keratectomy for myopia. *Refract Corneal Surg.* 1993;9(2suppl):S65.

Cavanaugh TB, Durrie DS, Riedel SM, et al. Centration of excimer laser photorefractive keratectomy relative to the pupil. *J Cataract Refract Surg.* 1993;19(Suppl):144.

Cavanaugh TB, Durrie DS, Riedel SM, et al. Topographical analysis of the centration of excimer laser photorefractive keratectomy. *J Cataract Refract Surg.* 1993;19(Suppl):136.

Cennamo G, Rosa N, Guida E, et al. Evaluation of corneal thickness and endothelial cells before and after excimer laser photorefractive keratectomy. *Refract Corneal Surg.* 1994;10:137.

Cennamo G, Rosa N, Guida E, Del Prete A, Sebastiani A. Evaluation of corneal thickness and endothelial cells before and after excimer laser photorefractive keratectomy. *J Refract Corneal Surg.* 1994;10(2):137-141.

Cherry PM. Removal of epithelium and scraping the underlying stroma as treatment for photorefractive keratectomy overcorrection or undercorrection of myopia. *Ophthalmic Surgery and Lasers.* 1996;27(5 Suppl):S487-S492.

Cherry PM. The treatment of pain following excimer laser photorefractive keratectomy: additive effect of local anesthetic drops, topical diclofenac, and bandage soft contact. *Ophthalmic Surgery and Lasers.* 1996;27(5 Suppl):S477-S480.

Cherry PMH, Tutton MK, Adhikary H, et al. The treatment of pain following photorefractive keratectomy. *Refract Corneal Surg.* 1994;10(2 Suppl):S222-225.

Cho YS, Kim CG, Kim WB, Kim CW. Multistep photorefractive keratectomy for high myopia. *Refract Corneal Surg.* 1993;9(Suppl):S37-S41.

Choyce DP. The correction of high myopia. *Refract Corneal Surg.* 1992;8:242.

Corbett MC, O'Brart DP, Marshall J. Do topical corticosteroids have a role following excimer laser photorefractive keratectomy? [see comments]. *J Refract Surg.* 1995;11(5):380-387. Review.

Corbett MC, O'Brart DP, Warburton FG, Marshall J. Biologic and environmental risk factors for regression after photorefractive keratectomy. *Ophthalmology.* 1996;103(9):1381-1391.

Corbett MC, Prydal JI, Verma S, Oliver KM, Pande M, Marshall J. An in vivo investigation of the structures responsible for corneal haze after photorefractive keratectomy and their effect on visual function. *Ophthalmology.* 1996;103(9):1366-1380.

Corbett MC, Verma S, O'Brart DP, Oliver KM, Heacock G, Marshall J. Effect of ablation profile on wound healing and visual performance 1 year after excimer laser photorefractive keratectomy. *Br J Ophthalmol.* 1996;80(3):224-234.

Dausch D, Klein R, Landesz M, Schroder E. Photorefractive keratectomy to correct astigmatism with myopia or hyperopia. *J Cataract Refract Surg.* 1994;20(Suppl):252-257

Dausch D, Klein R, Schroder E. Excimer laser photorefractive keratectomy for hyperopia. *Refract Corneal Surg.* 1993;9(1):20-28.

Demers P, Thompson P, Bernier RG, Lemire J, Laflamme P. Effect of occlusive pressure patching on the rate of epithelial wound healing after photorefractive keratectomy. *J Cataract Refract Surg.* 1996;22(1):59-62.

Ditzen K, Anschutz T, Schroder E. Photorefractive keratectomy to treat low, medium, and high myopia: a multicenter study. *J Cataract Refract Surg.* 1994;20 Suppl:234-238.

Dutt S, Steinert RF, Raizman MB, Puliafito CA. One-year results of excimer laser photorefractive keratectomy for low to moderate myopia. *Arch Ophthalmol.* 1994;112(11):1427-1436.

Ehlers N, Hjortdal JO. Excimer laser refractive keratectomy for high myopia. *Ophthalmologica.* 1992;70:578-586.

Englanoff JS, Kolahdouz-Isfahani AH, Moreira H, et al. In situ collagen gel mold as an aid in excimer laser superficial keratectomy. *Ophthalmology.* 1992;99(8):1201-1208.

Epstein D, Fagerholm P, Hamberg-Nystrom H, Tengroth B. Twenty-four-month follow-up of excimer laser photorefractive keratectomy for myopia. Refractive and visual acuity results. *Ophthalmology.* 1994;101(9):1558-1564. Discussion.

Epstein D, Tengroth B, Fagerholm P, Hamberg-Nystrom H. Excimer retreatment of regression after photorefractive keratectomy. *Am J Ophthalmology.* 1994;117(4):456-461.

Fagerholm P, Fitzsimmons TD, Orndahl M, et al. Phototherapeutic keratectomy: long-term results in 166 eyes. *Refract Corneal Surg.* 1993;9(Suppl):S76.

Fagerholm P, Hamberg-Nystrom H, Tengroth B, Epstein D. Effect of postoperative steroids on the refractive outcome of photorefractive keratectomy for myopia with the Summit excimer laser. *J Cataract Refract Surg.* 1994;20(Suppl):212-215.

Fichte CM, Bell AM. Ongoing results of excimer laser photorefractive keratectomy for myopia: subjective patient impressions. *J Cataract Refract Surg.* 1994;20(Suppl):268.

Fitzsimmons TD, Fagerholm P, Tengroth B. Steroid treatment of myopic regression: acute refractive and topographic changes in excimer photorefractive keratectomy patients. *Cornea.* 1993;12(4):358.

Forster W, Grewe S, Atzler U, et al. Phototherapeutic keratectomy in corneal diseases. *Refract Corneal Surg.* 1993;9(2suppl):S85.

Frangie JP, Park SB, Kim J, Aquavella JV. Excimer laser keratectomy after radial keratotomy. *Am J Ophthalmol.* 1993;115(5):634.

Gallinaro C, Toulemont PJ, Cochener B, Colin J. Excimer laser photorefractive keratectomy to correct astigmatism. *J Cataract Refract Surg.* 1996;22(5):557-563.

Gartry DS, Kerr-Muir MG, Lohmann CP, Marshall J. The effect of topical corticosteroids on refractive outcome and corneal haze after photorefractive keratectomy. A prospective, randomized, double-blind trial. *Arch Ophthalmol.* 1992;110(7):944-952.

Gartry DS, Kerr-Muir MG, Marshall J. Excimer laser photorefractive keratectomy: 18-month follow-up. *Ophthalmology.* 1992;99(8):1209-1219.

Gartry DS, Kerr-Muir MG, Marshall J. Photorefractive keratectomy with an argon-flouride excimer laser. A clinical study. *Refract Corneal Surg.* 1990;6:36-43.

Gebhardt BM, Salmeron B, McDonald MB. Effect of excimer laser energy on the growth potential of corneal keratocytes. *Cornea.* 1990;9(3):205.

Gimbel HV, DeBroff BM, Beldavs RA, van Westenbrugge JA, Ferensowicz M. Comparison of laser and manual removal of corneal epithelium for photorefractive keratectomy. *J Refract Surg.* 1995;11(1):36-41.

Gimbel HV, Van Westenbrugge JA, Johnson WH, et al. Visual, refractive, and patient satisfaction results following bilateral photorefractive keratectomy for myopia. *Refract Corneal Surg.* 1993;9(2suppl):S5-S10.

Goggin M, Foley-Nolan A, Algawi K, O'Keefe M. Regression after photorefractive keratectomy for myopia. *J Cataract Refract Surg.* 1996;22(2):194-196.

Goodman GL, Trokel SL, Stark WJ. Corneal healing following laser refractive keratectomy. *Arch Ophthalmol.* 1989;107:1799.

Gottsch JD, Gilbert ML, Goodman DF, et al. Excimer laser ablative treatment of microbial keratitis. *Ophthalmology.* 1991;98(2):146.

Hadden OB, Morris AT, Ring CP. Excimer laser surgery for myopia and myopic astigmatism. *Austral NZ J Ophthalmol.* 1995;23(3):183-188.

Hamberg-Nystrom H, Fagerholm P, Tengroth B, Sjoholm C. Thirty-six month follow-up of excimer laser photorefractive keratectomy for myopia. *Ophthalmic Surgery and Lasers.*1 996;27(5 Suppl):S418-S420

Hamberg-Nystrom H, Tengroth B, Fagerholm P, Epstein D, van der Kwast EM. Patient satisfaction following photorefractive keratectomy for myopia. *J Refract Surg.* 1995;11(3 Suppl):S335-336.

Hartstein J. Astigmatism and contact lenses. In: *Contemporary Contact Lens Practice.* St. Louis: CV Mosby; 1991.

Hecht J. These UV-range lasers are moving swiftly from laboratory experimentation to commercial products. *Lasers & Applications.* December 1983:238-244.

Heitzmann J, Binder PS, Kassar BS, Nordan LT. The correction of high myopia using the excimer laser. *Arch Ophthalmol.* 1993;111:1627-1634.

Hersh PS, Burnstein Y, Carr J, Etwaru G, Mayers M. Excimer laser phototherapeutic keratectomy. Surgical strategies and clinical outcomes. *Ophthalmology.* 1996;103(8):1210-1222.

Hjortdal JO, Bohm A, Kohlhaas M, et al. Mechanical stability of the cornea after radial keratotomy and photorefractive keratectomy. *J Refract Surg.* 1996;12(4):459-466.

Jardins SLL, Auclin F, Roman S, et al. Results of photorefractive keratectomy on 63 myopic eyes with six months minimum follow-up. *J Cataract Refract Surg.* 1994;20(Suppl):22.

Javitt JC, Chiang YP. *The socioeconomic aspects of laser refractive surgery.* Washington, DC: Georgetown University: 1993.

John ME, Martines E, Cvintal T, Ballew C. Excimer laser photoablation of primary familial amyloidosis of the cornea. *Refract Corneal Surg.* 1993;9(Suppl):S138.

Johnson DA, Haight DH, Kelly SE, et al. Reproducibility of videokeratographic digital subtraction maps after excimer laser photorefractive keratectomy. *Ophthalmology*. 1996;103(9):1392-1398.

Keats RH, Bloom RT, Ren Q, et al. Fibronectin on excimer laser and diamond knife incisions. *J Cataract Refract Surg*. 1989;15(4):404.

Kim JH, Hahn TW, Lee YC, Sah WJ. Clinical experience of two-step photorefractive keratectomy in 19 eyes with high myopia. *Refract Corneal Surg*. 1993;9(Suppl):S44-S47.

Kim JH, Hahn TW, Lee YC, Sah WJ. Excimer laser photorefractive keratectomy for myopia: two-year follow-up. *J Cataract Refract Surg*. 1994;20(Suppl):229-233.

Klyce SD, Smolek MK. Corneal topography of excimer laser photorefractive keratectomy. *Cataract Refract Surg*. 1993;19(Suppl):122.

Krueger RR, Campos M, Wang XW, et al. Corneal surface morphology following excimer laser ablation with humidified gases. *Arch Ophthalmol*. 1993;111(8):1131.

Krueger RR, Krasinski JS, Radzewicz C, et al. Photography of shock waves during excimer laser ablation of the cornea: effect of helium gas on propagation velocity. *Cornea*. 1993;12(4):330.

Krueger RR, Saedy NF, McDonnell PJ. Clinical analysis of steep central islands after excimer laser photorefractive keratectomy. *Arch Ophthalmol*. 1996;114(4):377-381.

Lang GK, Schroeder E, Koch JW, et al. Excimer laser keratoplasty. Part 1: basic concepts. *Ophthalmic Surg*. 1989;20(4):262.

Lang GK, Schroeder E, Koch JW, et al. Excimer laser keratoplasty. Part 2: elliptical keratoplasty. *Ophthalmic Surg*. 1989;20(5):342.

Lans LJ. Experimentelle unterschungen wber entstehung von astigmatissus durch niehte-performende corneawunden, Albert von Graefes. *Arch Ophthalmol*. 1988;45:117-152.

Lavery FL. Photorefractive keratectomy in 472 eyes. *Refract Corneal Surg*. 1993;9(Suppl):98-100.

L'Esperance FA. *Ophthalmic Lasers*. 3rd ed. 1989.

Lin DT. Corneal topographic analysis after excimer photorefractive keratectomy. *Ophthalmology*. 1994;101(8):1432-1439.

Lin DTC, Sutton HF, Berman M. Corneal topography following excimer photorefractive keratectomy for myopia. *J Cataract Refract Surg*. 1993;19(Suppl):149.

Lohmann CP, Fitzke F, O'Brart D, et al. Corneal light scattering and visual performance in myopic individuals with spectacles, contact lenses, or excimer laser photorefractive keratectomy. *Am J Ophthalmol*. 1993;115:444.

Lohmann CP, Fitzke FW, O'Brart D, Kerr-Muir M, Marshall J. Halos--a problem for all myopes? A comparison between spectacles, contact lenses, and photorefractive keratectomy. *Refract Corneal Surg*. 1993;9(2 Suppl):S72-75.

Lohmann CP, Timberlake GT, Fitzke FW, et al. Corneal light scattering after excimer laser photorefractive keratectomy: the objective measurements of haze. *Refract Corneal Surg*. 1992;8(2):114.

Machat JJ. Double-blind corticosteroid trial in identical twins following photorefractive keratectomy. *Refract Corneal Surg*. 1993;9(2suppl):S105.

Maguen E, Salz JJ, Nesburn AB, et al. Results of excimer laser photorefractive keratectomy for the correction of myopia. *Ophthalmology*. 1994;101(9):1548-1557. Discussion.

Maguire LJ, Zabel RW, Parker P, Lindstrom RL. Topography and raytracing analysis of patients with excellent visual acuity 3 months after excimer laser photorefractive keratectomy for myopia. *Refract Corneal Surg.* 1991;7:122.

Maloney RK. Corneal topography and optical zone location in photorefractive keratectomy. *Refract Corneal Surg.* 1990;6:363.

Mandell RB. Corneal power correction factor for photorefractive keratectomy. *Refract Corneal Surg.* 1994;10(Suppl):125.

Mardelli PG, Piebenga LW, Matta CS, Hyde LL, Gira J. Corneal endothelial status 12 to 55 months after excimer laser photorefractive keratectomy. *Ophthalmology*. 1995;102(4):544-549. Discussion.

McDonald M, et al. Excimer laser surface shaping of the primate cornea for the correction of myopia. *Invest Ophthalmol Vis Sci.* 1988;29:310.

McDonald MB, Frantz JM, Klyce SD, et al. Central photorefractive keratectomy for myopia: the blind eye study. *Arch Ophthalmol.* 1990;108(6):799.

McDonald MB, Kaufman HE, Frantz JM, et al. Excimer laser ablation in a human eye, case report. *Arch Ophthalmol.* 1989;107(5):641.

McDonald MB, Liu JC, Byrd T, et al. Central photorefractive keratectomy for myopia. Partially sighted and normally sighted eyes. *Ophthalmology*. 1991;98:1327-1358.

McDonnell PJ. Lans lecture: refractive surgery and your practice. *Refract Corneal Surg.* 1993;9:121.

McDonnell PJ, Garbus JJ, Salz JJ. Excimer laser myopic photorefractive keratectomy after undercorrected radial keratotomy. *Refract Corneal Surg.* 1991;7:146.

McDonnell PJ, Moreira H, Garbus J, et al. Photorefractive keratectomy to create toric ablations for correction of astigmatism. *Arch Ophthalmol.* 1991;109:710-713.

Meyer JC, Stulting RD, Thompson KP, Durrie DS. Late onset of corneal scar after excimer laser photorefractive keratectomy. *Am J Ophthalmol.* 1996;121(5):529-539.

Migden M, Elkins BS, Clinch TE. Phototherapeutic keratectomy for corneal scars. *Ophthalmic Surgery and Lasers.* 1996;27(5 Suppl):S503-S507.

Moreira H, Garbus JJ, Fasano A, et al. Multifocal corneal topographic changes with excimer laser photorefractive keratectomy. *Arch Ophthalmol.* 1992:110.

Morrow GL, Stein RM. Evaluation of corneal topography: past, present and future trends. *Can J Ophthalmol.* 1992;27:213.

Munnerlyn CR, Koons SJ, Marshall J. Photorefractive keratectomy: a technique for laser refractive surgery. *J Cataract Refract Surg.* 1988;14:46.

Neumann AC, Fyodorov S, Sanders DR. Radial thermokeratoplasty for the correction of hyperopia. *Refract Corneal Surg.* 1990;6:404-411.

Niesen UM, Businger U, Schipper I. Disability glare after excimer laser photorefractive keratectomy for myopia. *J Refract Surg.* 1996;12(2):S267-268.

O'Brart DP, Gartry DS, Lohmann CP, Muir MG, Marshall J. Excimer laser photorefractive keratectomy for myopia: comparison of 4.00- and 5.00-millimeter ablation zones. *J Refract Corneal Surg.* 1994;10(2):87-94.

O'Brart DP, Lohmann CP, Fitzke FW, Klonos G, Corbett MC, Kerr-Muir MG, Marshall J. Disturbances in night vision after excimer laser photorefractive keratectomy. *Eye.* 1994;8(Pt 1):46-51.

O'Brart DP, Lohmann CP, Fitzke FW, Smith SE, Kerr-Muir MG, Marshall J. Night vision after excimer laser photorefractive keratectomy: haze and halos. *Eur J Ophthalmology.* 1994;4(1):43-51.

O'Brart DP, Lohmann CP, Klonos G, et al. The effects of topical corticosteroids and plasmin inhibitors on refractive outcome, haze, and visual performance after photorefractive keratectomy. A prospective, randomized, observer-masked study. *Ophthalmology.* 1994;101(9):1565-1574.

Olson RJ. The altar of high technology and the excimer laser. *Arch Ophthalmol.* 1991;109(4):489.

Ozler SA, Liaw LH, Neev J, et al. Acute ultrastructural changes of cornea after excimer laser ablation. *Invest Ophthalmol Vis Sci.* 1992;33(3):540.

Paige N, Mustaler KL. Orthokeratology: a retrospective study. *Contact Lens Spectrum.* September 1986:24-26.

Pallikaris I, McDonald MB, Siganos D, et al. Tracker-assisted photorefractive keratectomy for myopia of -1 to -6 diopters. *J Refract Surg.* 1996;12(2):240-247.

Pallikaris IG, Siganos DS. Excimer laser in situ keratomileusis and photorefractive keratectomy for correction of high myopia. *J Refract Corneal Surg.* 1994;10(5):498-510.

Pavlin CJ, Harasiewicz K, Foster S. Ultrasound biomicroscopic assessment of the cornea following excimer laser photokeratectomy. *J Cataract Refract Surg.* 1994;20(Suppl):206.

Pender PM. Photorefractive keratectomy for myopic astigmatism: phase IIA of the Federal Drug Administration study (12 to 18 months follow-up). Excimer Laser Study Group. *J Cataract Refract Surg.* 1994;20 Suppl:262-264.

Phillips AF, Szerenyi K, Campos M, et al. Arachidonic acid metabolites after excimer laser corneal surgery. *Arch Ophthalmol.* 1993;111(9):1273.

Piebenga LW, Matta CS, Deitz MR, et al. Excimer photorefractive keratectomy for myopia. *Ophthalmology.* 1993;100(9):1335.

Pop M, Aras M. Multizone/multipass photorefractive keratectomy: six month results. *J Cataract Refract Surg.* 1995;21(6):633-643.

Puliafito CA, Steinert RF, Deutsch TF, et al. Excimer laser ablation of the cornea and lens: experimental studies. *Ophthalmology.* 1985;92:741-748.

Rabinowitz YS, McDonnell PJ. Identifying progression of subclinical keratoconus by serial topography analysis. *Am J Ophthalmol.* 1991;112:41-45

Rapuano CJ, Laibson PR. Excimer laser phototherapeutic keratectomy for anterior corneal pathology. *CLAO J.* 1994;20(4):253-257.

Ren Q, Simon G, Legeais JM, et al. Ultraviolet solid-state laser (213-nm) photorefractive keratectomy in vivo study. *Ophthalmology.* 1994;101(5):883.

Robin JB. Excimer laser corneal surgery. *Ophthalmology Clinics of North America.* 1990;3(4).

Salah T, Waring GO, El-Maghraby A, Moadel K, Grimm SB. Excimer laser in-situ keratomileusis (LASIK) under a corneal flap for myopia of 2 to 20 D. *Trans Amer Ophthalmol Soc.* 1995;93:163-183. Discussion. 1995;184-190.

Salah T, Waring GO, El-Maghraby A, Moadel K, Grimm SB. Excimer laser in situ keratomileusis under a corneal flap for myopia of 2 to 20 diopters [see comments]. *Am J Ophthalmol.* 1996;121(2):143-155.

Salz JJ, Maguen E, Nesburn AB, et al. A two-year experience with excimer laser photorefractive keratectomy for myopia. *Ophthalmology.* 1993;100(6):873-882.

Schein OD. Phototoxicity and the cornea. *J Natl Med Assoc.* 1992;84(7):579.

Schipper I, Senn P, Lechner A. Tapered transition zone and surface smoothing ameliorate the results of excimer-laser photorefractive keratectomy for myopia. *Ger J Ophthalmol.* 1996;4(6):368-373.

Seiler T, Bende T, Wollensak J. Excimer laser keratectomy for the correction of astigmatism. *Am J Ophthalmol.* 1988;105:117.

Seiler T, Genth U, Holschbach A, Derse M. Aspheric photorefractive keratectomy with excimer laser. *Refract Corneal Surg.* 1993;9(3):166.\

Seiler T, Holschbach A, Derse M, et al. Complications of myopic photorefractive keratectomy with excimer laser. *Ophthalmology.* 1994;101(1):154.

Seiler T, Matallana M, Bende T. Laser thermokeratoplasty by means of a pulsed holmium:YAG laser for hyperopic correction. *Refract Corneal Surg.* 1990;6(5):335-339.

Seiler T, Reckmann W, Maloney RK. Effective spherical aberration of the cornea as a quantitative descriptor in corneal topography. *J Cataract Refract Surg.* 1993;19(Suppl):155.

Seiler T, Wollensak J. Myopic photorefractive keratectomy with the excimer laser. One year follow-up. *Ophthalmology.* 1991;98:1157-1163.

Shah SI, Hersh PS. Photorefractive keratectomy for myopia with a 6-mm beam diameter. *J Refract Surg.* 1996;12(3):341-346.

Sher NA, Barak M, Daya S, et al. Excimer laser photorefractive keratectomy in high myopia: a multicenter study. *Arch Ophthalmol.* 1992;110:935-942.

Sher NA, Bowers RA, Zabel RW, et al. Clinical use of the 193-nm excimer laser in the treatment of corneal scars. *Arch Ophthalmol.* 1991;109:491.

Sher NA, Chen V, Bowers RA, et al. The use of the 193 nm laser for myopic photorefractive keratectomy in sighted eyes: a multicenter study. *Arch Ophthalmol.* 1991;109:1525-1530.

Sher NA, Hardten DR, DeMarchi J, Lindstrom RL. Excimer photorefractive keratectomy in very high myopia. *Seminars in Ophthalmology.* 1994;9(2):97-101.

Sher NA, Hardten DR, Fundingsland B, DeMarchi J, Carpel E, Doughman DJ, Lane SS, Ostrov C, Eiferman R, Frantz JM, et al. 193-nm excimer photorefractive keratectomy in high myopia. *Ophthalmology.* 1994;101(9):1575-1582.

Shimizu K, Amano S, Tanaka S. Photorefractive keratectomy for myopia: one-year follow-up in 97 eyes. *Refract Corneal Surg.* 1994;10(Suppl):S178.

Spadea L, Sabetti L, Balestrazzi E. Effect of centering excimer laser PRK on refractive results: a corneal topography study. *Refract Corneal Surg.* 1993;9(Suppl).

Sperduto RD, Seigel D, Roberts J, Rowland M. Prevalence of myopia in the United States. *Arch Ophthalmol.* 1983;101:405.

Spigelman AV, Albert WC, Cozean CH, et al. Treatment of myopic astigmatism with the 193 nm excimer laser utilizing aperture elements. *J Cataract Refract Surg.* 1994;20(Suppl):258-261.

Srinivasan R, Mayne-Banton V. Self-developing photoetching of poly(ethylene terephthalate) films by far UV excimer laser radiation. *Appl Phys Lett.* 1982;41:576.

Stein HA, Slatt BJ, Stein RM. Fitting guide for rigid and soft contact lenses. *A Practical Approach Textbook.* 3rd ed. 1990.

Stein HA, Slatt BJ, Stein RM. *Refractive Surgery. The Ophthalmic Assistant.* St. Louis, MO: CV Mosby Co; 1994:651.

Stein R. *Laser-PRK.* Toronto, Canada:Beacon Eye Institute: 34-53.

Stein R. Ophthalmologists need to understand preoperative assessments, techniques, and postoperative management to achieve satisfactory visual outcomes. *OSN.* 1996;Sept 15:38.

Stein R. Quick epithelial removal key to good outcomes. *OSN.* 1996;May 15:33.

Stein R, Stein HA, Cheskes A, Symons S. Photorefractive keratectomy and postoperative pain. *Am J Ophthalmol.* 1994;117(3):403-405.

Steinert RF, Puliafito CA. Corneal incisions with the excimer laser. In: Sanders DR, Hoffman RF, Salz JJ, eds. *Refractive Corneal Surgery.* Thorofare, NJ: SLACK, Inc; 1986.

Steinert RF, Puliafito CA. Excimer laser phototherapeutic keratectomy for a corneal nodule. *Refract Corneal Surg.* 1991;6:352.

Stulting RD, Thompson KP, Waring GO, Lynn M. The effect of photorefractive keratectomy on the corneal endothelium. *Ophthalmology.* 1996;103(9):1357-1365.

Tabaoda J, Mikesell GW, Reed RD. Response of the corneal epithelium to KrF excimer laser pulses. *Health Phys.* 1981;40:766.

Talley AR, Hardten DR, Sher NA, et al. Results one year after using the 193-nm excimer laser for photorefractive keratectomy in mild to moderate myopia. *Am J Ophthalmol.* 1994;118(3):304-311.

Talley AR, Sher NA, Kim MS, et al. Use of the 193 nm excimer laser for photorefractive keratectomy in low to moderate myopia. *J Cataract Refract Surg.* 1994;20(Suppl):239-242.

Taylor HR, Kelly P, Alpins N. Excimer laser correction of myopic astigmatism. *J Cataract Refract Surg.* 1994;20(Suppl):243-251.

Teal P, Breslin C, Arshinoff S, Edmison D. Corneal subepithelial infiltrates following excimer laser photorefractive keratectomy. *J Cataract Refract Surg.* 1995;21(5):516-518.

Tengroth B, Epstein D, Fagerholm P, et al. *Ophthalmology.* 1993;100:739-745.

Thompson FB, McDonnell PJ. *Color Atlas/Textbook of Excimer Laser Surgery.* New York, NY: Igaku-Shoin Medical Publishers; 1993:158.

Thompson KP, Barraquer E, Parel JM, et al. Potential use of lasers for penetrating keratoplasty. *J Cataract Refract Surg.* 1989;15(4):397.

Thompson V, Durrie DS, Cavanaugh TB. Philosophy and technique for excimer laser phototherapeutic keratectomy. *Refract Corneal Surg.* 1993;9(Suppl):S81.

Thompson VM, Seiler T, Durrie D, Cavanaugh TB. Holmium:YAG laser thermokeratoplasty for hyperopia and astigmatism: an overview. *Refract Corneal Surg.* 1993;9(Suppl):S134-S137.

Thornton SP. *Radial and Astigmatic Keratotomy.* Thorofare, NJ: SLACK, Inc; 1994:204.

Trocme SD, Mack KA, Gill KS, Gold DH, Milstein BA, Bourne WM. Central and peripheral endothelial cell changes after excimer laser photorefractive keratectomy for myopia. *Arch Ophthalmol.* 1996;114(8):925-928.

Trokel SL. Development of the excimer laser in ophthalmology: a personal perspective. *Refract Corneal Surg.* 1990;6(5):357.

Trokel SL. Evolution of excimer laser corneal surgery. *J Cataract Refract Surg.* 1989;15:373.

Trokel SL, Srinivasan R, Braren B. Excimer laser surgery of the cornea. *Am J Ophthalmol.* 1983;96:710.

Tsubota K, Toda I, Itoh S. Reduction of subepithelial haze after photorefractive keratectomy by cooling the cornea. *Am J Ophthalmology.* 1993;115(6):820-821. Letter.

Tutton MK, Cherry PM, Raj PS, Fsadni MG. Efficacy and safety of topical diclofenac in reducing ocular pain after excimer photorefractive keratectomy. *J Cataract Refract Surg.* 1996;22(5):536-541.

Verma S, Marshall J. Control of pain after photorefractive keratectomy. *J Refract Surg.* 1996;12(3):358-364. Review.

Waring GO. FDA panel recommends conditional approval of excimer laser phototherapeutic keratectomy (PTK) [news]. *J Refract Cataract Surg.* 1994;10(2):77-78.

Waring GO III. *Refractive Keratotomy for Myopia and Astigmatism.* Mosby-Year Book, Inc; 1992:1326. (PTK) [news].

Waring GO III, Lynn ML, Culbertson W, et al. Three year results of the prospective evaluation of radial keratotomy (PERK) study. *Ophthalmology.* 1987;94:1339-1354.

Weinstock SJ. Excimer laser keratectomy: one year results with 100 myopic patients. *CLAO J.* 1993;19(3):178.

Weinstock SJ, Machat JJ. Excimer laser keratectomy for the correction of myopia. *CLAO J.* 1993;19(2):133.

Werblin TP, Kaufman HE. Epikeratophakia: the surgical correction of aphakia. Preliminary results in a non-human primate model. *Eur Eye Research.* 1981;1:131-137.

Wilson SE, Klyce SD. Advances in the analysis of corneal topography. *Surv Ophthalmol.* 1991;35(4).

Wilson SE, Klyce SD, McDonald MB, et al. Changes in corneal topography after excimer laser photorefractive keratectomy for myopia. *Ophthalmology.* 1991;98(9):1338.

Index

absorption, defined, 217

acuity, changing, after excimer laser treatment, 44-45

advertising, in excimer laser marketing, 198

Aesculap-Meditec
    address, phone, 213
    GmbH, address, phone, 213
    MEL-60, 14, 18-21
    MEL-70, 14, 18-21

age, patient selection and, 31-32

ALK, defined, 217

arcuate haze, as complication, 147-150

astigmatism, 111-115, 185
    congenital myopic astigmatism, 113
    indications, 113-114
    postoperative astigmatism, 113
    postoperative management, 114
    radial keratotomy, photorefractive keratectomy, compared, 166
    surgical technique, 113-114
    technical operation, 111-113
    transverse keratotomy for astigmatism, 185

atom, defined, 217

audience, target, identifying, 196-197

Autonomous Technologies
    address, phone, 213
    T-PRK, 14, 21-25

Avco Everett Research Laboratory, 7

Averos, Guillimero, laser assisted in situ keratomileusis, 172

avocation, patient selection and, 34

Barraquer, Jose, laser assisted in situ keratomileusis, 172

benefits, excimer laser treatment, 37-41

brightness, laser light, 3

broad beam lasers. See wide field laser

Buratto, Lucio, laser assisted in situ keratomileusis, 172

central islands
    as complication, 143-145

retreatment and, 157

Chiron Vision
    address, phone, 213
    Keracor 116, 14-18
    Keracor 117, 14-18
    Technolas 217 C-LASIK, 14

coherence
    defined, 217
    laser light, 3-4

Coherent Medical
    address, phone, 213
    Schwind Keratom, 14-18

computerized videokeratography, patient selection and, 34

contraindications, 35-36
    ocular pathologies, 35
    refraction anomalies, 35-36
    systemic pathologies, 35

corneal haze, retreatment and, 156

corneal infection, as complication, 139-140

corticosteroid use, side effects of, 138

cost, radial keratotomy, photorefractive keratectomy, compared, 166

decentered ablations, retreatment and, 156-157

decentration, as complication, 145

degree of correction, radial keratotomy, photorefractive keratectomy, compared, 165

delayed epithelial healing, as complication, 140-141

diffuse haze, as complication, 146-147

dimer, defined, 217

directionality, laser light, 4

discomfort, as complication, 139

discussions with patient
    operative, 44
    postoperative, 44-45
    preoperative, 43-44

early complications, 139-146

electromagnetic spectrum, defined, 217